Preventing Diabetes

Preventing Diabetes

Theory, Practice and New Approaches

DAN MIRCEA CHEŢA, MD, PhD

Carol Davila University of Medicine and Pharmacy
and N. Paulescu Institute of Nutrition and Metabolic Diseases,
Bucharest, Romania

JOHN WILEY & SONS, LTD
Chichester • New York • Weinheim • Brisbane • Singapore • Toronto

National   01243 779777
International (+44) 1243 779777
e-mail (for orders and customer service enquiries): cs-books@wiley.co.uk
Visit our Home Page on http://www.wiley.co.uk
            or http://www.wiley.com

Other Wiley Editorial Offices

John Wiley & Sons, Inc., 605 Third Avenue,
New York, NY 10158-0012, USA

WILEY-VCH Verlag GmbH, Pappelallee 3,
D-69469 Weinheim, Germany

Jacaranda Wiley Ltd, 33 Park Road Milton,
Queensland 4064, Australia

John Wiley & Sons (Asia) Pte Ltd, 2 Clementi Loop #02-01,
Jim Xing Distripark, Singapore 129809

John Wiley & Sons (Canada) Ltd, 22 Worcester Road,
Rexdale, Ontario M9W 1L1, Canada

Library of Congress Cataloging-in-Publication Data
Cheţa, Dan.
    Preventing diabetes : theory, practice, and new approaches   /   Dan Mircea Cheţa.
        p. cm.
    Includes bibliographical references and index.
    ISBN 0-471-99914-8 (cased   :   alk. paper)
    1. Diabetes—Prevention.   I. Title.
    [DNLM: 1. Diabetes Mellitus—prevention & control.   WK 810 C526p 1999]
RA645.D5C48   1999
616.4'6205—dc21
DNLM/DLC   99-14789
for Library of Congress   CIP

British Library Cataloguing in Publication Data

A catalogue record for this book is available from the British Library

ISBN 0-471-99914-8

Typeset in 11/13pt Palatino from the author's disks by Techset Composition Ltd, Salisbury.
Printed and bound in Great Britain by Biddles Ltd, Guildford and King's Lynn.
This book is printed on acid-free paper responsibly manufactured from sustainable forestry, in which at least two trees are planted for each one used for paper production.

Contents

Foreword

During the last 15 years, the picture of diabetes mellitus has changed dramatically as a consequence of the numerous pieces of information generated by the constantly growing research in this field. New fundamental discoveries on the pathogenesis of both type 1 and 2 diabetes mellitus have led to the formulation of a series of scientific hypotheses that not only involve basic research but have also been used to develop novel strategies of therapy and prevention. New techniques in molecular biology have enabled identification and molecular cloning of crucial target proteins and uncovered the complexity of the genetic background involved in predisposition to disease. Also, thanks to animal models of the disease, diabetes mellitus is today one of the most intensely and actively researched medical subjects. Basic and clinical studies have unravelled the existence of new forms of diabetes mellitus, for instance latent autoimmune diabetes of the adult (LADA). The results of large clinical studies (DCCT, UKPDS, Stockholm Study and others) and the formulation of new hypoglycemic agents and new insulin preparations are rapidly changing the clinical picture of diabetes mellitus.

The increasing specialization of diabetes research is generating a wide gap between clinical diabetology and basic research. Thus, there is a growing need for books summarizing the most recent scientific discoveries and discussing new strategies to be applied in the everyday clinical management of people with diabetes. This is especially true when referring to the most controversial and demanding topic of diabetes research: primary and secondary prevention.

This book is an admirable example of a work edited by a true expert in both clinical diabetes and basic research and is aimed at bridging the gap between scientific theories and clinical application. The first part discusses the complex problem of the classification of diabetes mellitus in all its controversial aspects. Discussion of the major pathogenic theories, supported by the most relevant experimental data, then paves the way to the final analysis of the prevention strategies, which are simply but exhaustively presented in both their experimental bases and the practical application in clinical trials. The reference to the ongoing clinical studies of prevention of type 1 diabetes updates the reader in one of the more complex problems of modern diabetology.

The lucidity of the descriptions and the completeness of the work make this book a valuable reference text not only for the clinical diabetologist but for anyone who is seriously interested in the progresses of diabetes research.

Paolo Brunetti
Perugia, Italy

Acknowledgements

A long and fruitful collaboration with the teams led by Professors Paolo Brunetti of Perugia, Italy and Merl Arthur Charles of Irvine, California, USA, was of great help in the production of several chapters of this book. Recently, a cordial relationship has been established with Dr Pierre Thibert and his colleagues of the Sir Frederick Banting Research Centre in Ottawa, Canada, as well as with Dr Dennis L. Guberski and his colleagues at the University of Massachusetts, Worcester, USA.

The Romanian Academy of Medicine—especially its Secretary General, Professor Mihai Zamfirescu—encouraged both the research regarding the prevention of diabetes and the preparation of this text.

Dr Lawrence Chukwudi Nwabudike was of great assistance in the production of the English version. Dr Bogdan Orăşanu deserves thanks for his help in gathering references while my gratitude flows to Mădălina Andronescu, RN, for her secretarial assistance.

An atmosphere of cooperation with John Wiley & Sons prevailed during the entire period of writing and editing this book.

Introduction

Prevention is better than cure

Erasmus

Diabetes mellitus is one of the major public health problems of the transition period between the 20th and 21st centuries.

First, there is a dramatic increase in the frequency of the disease. An analysis of the epidemiologic data from the World Health Organization, the International Diabetes Federation and many other prestigious research groups showed that, in 1992, there were an estimated 100 million diabetic persons worldwide. In the year 2000, this figure is expected to rise to over 150 million and may attain 300 million by the year 2025[1–9] (Table I.1 and Figure I.1). At the time of the writing of this text it is almost certain that the figure of 130 million has already been exceeded.

The great majority (88–90%) are patients with type 2 diabetes (non-insulin-dependent diabetes mellitus; NIDDM). Without going into much detail, it should be interesting to underline the fact that the prevalence of NIDDM differs greatly with ethnic origin, from below 1% in some population groups in Africa, Asia and Latin America to 50% in the Pima Indians and to over 40% in the Nauruans (Micronesians). An important point for the future direction of medical policies is that if one takes an arbitrary point of 10% above which diabetes in adults can be considered frequent, only in the developing

Table I.1. The progressive increase in the frequency of diabetes mellitus at the end of the 20th century and the beginning of the 21st century

Year	Number of diabetic persons (millions)
1992	100
1994	110
1998	140
2000	Over 150
2010	235–240
2025	Over 250
2025–2030	Approximately 300 (other estimates)

Adapted from WHO, IDF and other epidemiologic sources

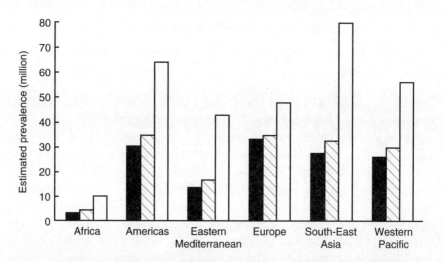

Figure I.1. WHO regional estimates of diabetes mellitus, 1995 (■), 2000 (▧) and 2025 (□). Adapted from reference 9

countries and the immigrant and minority communities of the developed nations is this limit exceeded. Almost 75% of all diabetic patients will be found in the developing countries in 2025[2]. This tendency has been clearly confirmed in the 1997 World Health Report[7].

Referring briefly to type 1 diabetes (insulin-dependent diabetes mellitus; IDDM), marked ethnic and geographic differences also exist. Thus, IDDM is one of the few chronic diseases where a 300-fold difference in risk has been noted. The place where a child lives is one of the most potent factors for the disease[3].

A second aspect that must be emphasized is that of the devastating complications of diabetes. Murray and Lopez of the WHO, for example, estimated a total number of 1 million cases of diabetic foot, 24 million cases of diabetic neuropathy, 6 million cases of amputation due to diabetes and 5 million cases of diabetic retino-pathy[10,11]. Cardiovascular complications (myocardial ischemia, stroke, peripheral vascular disease) are a major source of morbidity and mortality for individuals with diabetes; in the USA in 1992, almost 60% of deaths in people with diabetes were due to cardiovas-cular causes[6,12]. Murray and Lopez estimate a total of 3.8 million disability-adjusted life years (DALY) in 1990, a figure which is expected to increase to 9.5–15 million DALY in 2020. That means a twofold to fourfold increase in the burden of diabetes in this 30-year period[10,11]. The accurate evaluation of mortality due to diabetes is still difficult to achieve in many countries.

The huge costs of diabetes are another problem of top priority. Studies dedicated to these are increasing worldwide and their conclu-sions suffice to increase worry. Fox *et al.*, for example, estimated that the total costs of diabetes in the USA were about $91.8 billion dollars in 1992: of these $45.2 billion (49%) are direct costs and $46.6 billion (51%) are indirect costs[13]. Utilizing another method of evaluation, Rubin *et al.* noted that the healthcare costs of diabetes were $105.2 billion in 1992[14]. Both studies suggest that the cost of diabetes may be substantially higher than previously thought[15]. The total healthcare burden for Australia in 1989 was estimated at over A$375 million (US$267 million) for diabetes[16]. Selby *et al.* noted that diabetes is a costly disorder by virtue of its high prevalence and high per person costs. A large proportion of these costs are related to treating the complications of diabetes[17]. It is impossible at the moment to calculate the true global costs of diabetes but it is certainly astronomic. On the other hand, it must be emphasized that recent analyses of the costs and benefits of the intensive treatment of diabetes predict that morbidity and mortality can be drastically reduced. The overall cost-effectiveness is approximately the same for both type 1 and type 2 diabetes and is in the range of interventions that have historically been considered highly cost-effective[18].

The failure to diagnose diabetes before typical manifestations and complications occur is considered another problem of special importance. Half of the estimated 16 million Americans with diabetes are undiagnosed. The existence of diabetes is frequently not discovered until another medical problem occurs and hyperglycemia is found incidentally. It is critical that diabetes is diagnosed as soon as possible because diabetic complications frequently appear before diagnosis is made (in type 2 diabetes)[19]. At the time of diagnosis, about 20% of these patients have background retinopathy, 10–20% have microalbuminuria and 3–5% have neuropathy[18,19].

Another aspect that deserves mention is one that is "purely medical". The dramatic increase in diabetes and its complications has not received an adequate response from the public health services except in some areas. The medical world was to some extent surprised by the "phenomenon of diabetes mellitus" and has not yet adapted to its demands. There are not enough qualified medical personnel, there are not enough diabetes centers and there are not enough therapeutic resources. On the other hand, medical education at all levels does not accord sufficient importance to diabetes or to metabolic and nutritional problems in general. Romania, the country of origin of this work, recognizes a separate medical specialty, designated Diabetes, Nutrition and Metabolic Diseases, as a distinct specialty with a medical network specialized in this field. Nevertheless, the fight against diabetes and its complications has not attained to a high level and is beset with many hindrances.

If diabetes mellitus is such a serious threat to public health and—in general—for the development of human society, the increasingly decisive tendency to prediction and prevention is quite natural.

In the period 16–20 November 1992, the WHO Study Group on Prevention of Diabetes Mellitus comprising notable personalities of international diabetology held a reunion in Geneva. They produced a remarkable report entitled *Prevention of Diabetes Mellitus*, published in 1994[20]. Another memorable moment was the First World Congress on the Prevention of Diabetes and its Complications (Lyngby, Denmark, 1996). The second congress will take place in Slovenia in November 1999. The literature dedicated to this subject has increased considerably and, perhaps more importantly, the programs dedicated to the research into and the putting into practice of some methods for the prophylaxis of diabetes have grown in number.

The general strategies for the prevention of diabetes and its complications were well defined by the WHO report in 1994 (Table I.2). Three levels of prevention can be briefly classified:

- Primary prevention includes measures aimed at preventing the occurrence of the disease in susceptible subjects or populations through modifications of either environmental and behavioral risk factors or determinants or through specific interventions for susceptible individuals. Thus, primary prevention may have a population-based character or may be individualized for those with an increased risk for the development of the disease.
- Secondary prevention includes activities aimed at early diabetes as well as prompt and effective management to reverse the condition and/or halt its progression. An example is screening, which can be targeted at populations or high-risk subjects.
- Tertiary prevention is aimed at preventing the complications and disability that occur due to diabetes i.e. to prevent or delay the negative health consequences of diabetes in those who have already developed the disease. In Table I.2 the three successive stages of tertiary prevention are mentioned[20].

Works that deal with the analysis of strategies as well as the financial aspects of prediction and prevention of diabetes mellitus are of special importance[21–24].

Table I.2. General strategy for the prevention of diabetes mellitus and its complications

---

Primary prevention
- The population approach
- The high-risk approach

Secondary prevention

Tertiary prevention
- Prevention of the development of complications
- Prevention of the progression of complications to overt organ or tissue diseases
- Prevention of disability due to organ or tissue failure

Adapted from reference 20

Nevertheless, although there appears to be great promise, the field of prevention of diabetes mellitus and its complications is still far from effective[2]. Epidemiologic, economic and medicosocial data—some of which have been mentioned above—confirm, unfortunately, the precarious state of this field.

This modest work is dedicated to some aspects of the primary prevention of diabetes. Data and concepts from international literature will be presented in as coherent a form as possible with the addition of some personal results and opinions. Some practical suggestions will also be made. The fundamental purpose of a work such as this is to awaken as broad an interest as possible in the prevention of diabetes and to stimulate concrete preoccupation with this field. I do not believe that I am exaggerating when I assert that the prophylaxis of diabetes and its complications is an urgent requirement for medicine at the end of this century.

REFERENCES

1. McCarty D, Zimmet P. *Diabetes 1994 to 2010: Global Estimates and Projections.* Melbourne: International Diabetes Institute, 1994.
2. King H. Diabetes Mellitus: a growing international health care problem. *Intern Diabet Monit* 1997; **9**: 1–6.
3. Sekikawa A, LaPorte RE. Epidemiology of Insulin Dependent Diabetes Mellitus. In Alberti KGMM, Zimmet P, DeFronzo RA, Keen H (eds). *International Textbook of Diabetes Mellitus,* 2nd edn. Chichester: Wiley, 1997, 89–96.
4. Valle T, Tuomilehto J, Eriksson J. Epidemiology of NIDDM in Europids. In Alberti KGMM, Zimmet P, DeFronzo RA, Keen H (eds). *International Textbook of Diabetes Mellitus,* 2nd edn. Chichester: Wiley, 1997, 125–42.
5. De Courten M, Bennett PH, Tuomilehto J, Zimmet P. Epidemiology of NIDDM in Non-Europids. In Alberti KGMM, Zimmet P, DeFronzo RA, Keen H (eds). *International Textbook of Diabetes Mellitus,* 2nd edn. Chichester: Wiley, 1997, 143–70.
6. Keen H. Prevention of NIDDM. Slide Lecture Kit. UK: Medical Action Communications Ltd, 1995.
7. World Health Report 1997. *Conquering Suffering, Enriching Humanity.* Geneva: World Health Organization, 1997.

8. Jervell J. Why is Type 2 diabetes (NIDDM) becoming so common in developing countries? *IDF Bull* 1998; **43**(2): 6–7.

9. King H. The World Health Organization: An essential partner. *IDF Bull* 1998; **43**(3): 13–16.

10. Murray CJL, Lopez AD. *Global Health Statistics*. Geneva: World Health Organization, 1996.

11. Murray CJL, Lopez AD. *The Global Burden of Disease*. Geneva: World Health Organization, 1996.

12. American Diabetes Association. *Direct and Indirect Costs of Diabetes in the USA in 1992*. Alexandria, VA: American Diabetes Association, 1993.

13. Fox NA, Wills S, Thamer M. *Direct and Indirect Costs of Diabetes in the United States in 1992*. Alexandria VA: American Diabetes Association, 1993.

14. Rubin RJ, Altman WM, Mendelson DN. Health Care Expenditures for People with Diabetes Mellitus in 1992. *J Clin Endocrinol Metab* 1994; **78**: 809A–F.

15. Songer TJ. The Economics of Diabetes Care: USA. In Alberti KGMM, Zimmet P, DeFronzo RA, Keen H (eds). *International Textbook of Diabetes Mellitus*, 2nd edn. Chichester: Wiley, 1997, 1761–72.

16. Segal L, Carter R. The Economics of Diabetes Care: Australia. In Alberti KGMM, Zimmet P, DeFronzo RA, Keen H (eds). *International Textbook of Diabetes Mellitus*, 2nd edn. Chichester: Wiley, 1997, 1779–86.

17. Selby JV, Ray GT, Zhang D, Colby CJ. Excess Costs of Medical Care for Patients with Diabetes in a Managed Care Population. *Diabetes Care* 1997; **20**: 1396–1402.

18. Eastmann RC. Aspects of the health economics of diabetes intervention. *Intern Diabet Monit* 1997; **9**: 1–5.

19. Levetan CS, Passaro M, Jablonski K, Kass M, Ratner RE. Unrecognized diabetes among hospitalised patients. *Diabetes Care* 1998; **21**: 246–9.

20. *WHO Prevention of Diabetes Mellitus. Report of a WHO Study Group*. Geneva: World Health Organization, 1994.

21. Eastman RC, Javitt JJ, Herman WH *et al*. Prevention Strategies for Non-insulin Dependent Diabetes Mellitus: An Economic Perspective. In LeRoith D, Taylor SI, Olefsky JM (eds). *Diabetes Mellitus: A Fundamental and Clinical Text*. New York: Lippincott-Raven, 1996; 621–30.

22. *Costing Diabetes: The Case for Prevention*. Brussels: International Diabetes Federation, 1997.

23. *The Economics of Diabetes and Diabetes Care. A Report of the Diabetes Health Economics Study Group*. Brussels: International Diabetes Federation, 1997.

24. Hahl J, Simell T, Ilonen J, Knip M, Simell O. Costs of predicting IDDM. *Diabetologia* 1998; **41**: 79–85.

1

Difficulties Associated with the Classification of the Diabetic Syndrome

Both the treatment and the prevention of a disease (or of a syndrome) are strongly influenced by its diagnostic criteria and the classification of that disease (or syndrome). A clear, simple and unanimously accepted classification aids the development of precise methods of treatment. It also provides a valuable basis for the perfection of a truly efficient preventive strategy.

The complexity of the etiopathogenesis of diabetes mellitus has for a long time impeded the development of an adequate classification[1,2]. WHO experts have made considerable efforts in this field, producing many technical reports, and a new one is in the offing[3-5].

1.1 THE WHO CLASSIFICATION 13 YEARS AFTER ITS RELEASE

The specialist literature and the majority of diabetologists still work with the classification proposed by the WHO in 1985[4] (Table 1.1). This classification has a number of incontestable merits.

Thus, for example, the definition and clear separation of IDDM and NIDDM has become a major advantage for medical practice. The

Table 1.1. Present classification of diabetes mellitus and of other categories of glucose intolerance

---

A. Clinical classes

Diabetes mellitus (DM):
- Insulin-dependent diabetes mellitus (IDDM)
- Non-insulin-dependent diabetes mellitus (NIDDM):
  a) Non-obese
  b) Obese
- Malnutrition-related diabetes mellitus (MRDM)
- Other types of diabetes (associated with certain conditions and syndromes):
  1. Pancreatic disease
  2. Disease of hormonal etiology
  3. Drug-induced or chemical-induced conditions
  4. Abnormalities of insulin or its receptors
  5. Certain genetic syndromes
  6. Miscellaneous

Impaired glucose tolerance (IGT):
  a) Non-obese
  b) Obese
  c) Associated with certain conditions and syndromes

Gestational diabetes mellitus (GDM)

B. Statistical risk classes (subjects with normal glucose tolerance but increased risk of developing diabetes)

Previous abnormality of glucose tolerance
Potential abnormality of glucose tolerance

Adapted from Reference 4

ambiguity and useless details of the old classifications (such as that connected with the age of onset) have been eliminated. Although the terms "type 1 diabetes" and "type 2 diabetes" were not included in the WHO table and there have been some problems related to terminology, it has been recommended that these terms should be regarded as synonymous with IDDM and NIDDM respectively[4].

The recognition and definition of malnutrition-related diabetes mellitus (MRDM) and of gestational diabetes mellitus (GDM) also represented significant progress. I also believe that the precise enumeration of the entities included under the heading "Other types of diabetes" were beneficial.

Unfortunately, this classification presents a series of debatable aspects or eludes certain important issues. One of the criticisms is related to the obstinacy with which the term "diabetes" is avoided for the preclinical or secondary forms of the disease. The authors of the WHO reports have tried to justify this orientation but the solutions proposed are not convincing. The old staging of the progression of the disease (prediabetes or potential diabetes; latent diabetes; chemical diabetes; overt clinical diabetes) had the advantage of bringing the unity of diabetogenic processes to light even if the preliminary stages had a greater or lesser degree of instability. The preliminary stages may evolve progressively but may also be reversible. For the preventive actions (especially for the motivation of the subjects involved) we have to recognize that the old terminology was clearer and more useful. Terms such as "previous abnormality of glucose tolerance", "potential abnormality of glucose tolerance" and even "impaired glucose tolerance (IGT)" are difficult for the non-medical public to understand—and the expression "other types of diabetes associated with certain conditions and syndromes" refers in fact to secondary diabetes.

Another weakness of this classification appears to be the ignoring of those cases of diabetes which could not be included with precision either in type 1 diabetes or type 2 diabetes. The authors of the WHO report of 1985 were content to state that a separate class of "questionable insulin dependency" may be used, but this is not included in the classification because it cannot be clearly defined[4]. If this class involved only a small number of cases, perhaps things would have continued this way but, unfortunately, in diabetologic practice we frequently encounter this type of patient. There are diabetic centers which report a disturbing phenomenon—of the total number of patients treated with insulin the frequency of those with "questionable insulin deficiency" may be greater than that of those with IDDM[6,7]. Other studies suggest as many as 20% of patients who present initially with NIDDM may have slowly progressive IDDM[8,9]. I believe that this subject deserves to be treated in a separate section.

1.2 WHAT LIES BETWEEN IDDM AND NIDDM?

In an effort to appreciate the epidemiologic dimensions and principal clinical aspects of the so-called "questionable insulin dependency", I carried out a study of patients registered at the Diabetes Center in Bucharest (Romania) in 1984 and re-evaluated them 10 years later. As can be observed in Table 1.2, 971 cases were recorded in 1984. Initially, 32.44% of these received only dietary treatment, 60.56% received oral drugs and 7% received insulin. Ten years later, the therapeutic status of those still under study (723 patients) was as follows: 12.05% were still on diet as the sole therapy, 73.22% received oral medication, 14.73% received insulin. Note the reduction by almost two-thirds of the number of those treated by diet alone and the doubling of the proportion of those treated with insulin; the percentage of those treated with oral drugs rose by almost 13%.

Table 1.3 presents the situation of those patients (819; 84.35% of the total) who did not receive insulin therapy during the observation period. A huge decrease in the number of those treated with diet only

Table 1.2. General features of the diabetic patients (registered in Bucharest 1984)

Parameters	Initial	After 10 years**
Total no.: 971		
Sex: male 485 (49.85%)		
female 486 (50.05%)		
Mean age: 54.39 ± 13.27 years		
Pre-diagnosis period: 16.58 ± 34.37 months*		
Diabetes heredity: 14.62%*		
BMI	28.38 ± 13.78	27.95 ± 5.12
Glycemia (mg%)	180.40 ± 68.37	180.80 ± 62.78
Glycosuria (g/l)	21.05 ± 17.76	17.38 ± 16.47
Type of treatment (%):		
Diet (only)	32.44	12.05
Oral drugs	60.56	73.22
Insulin	7.00	14.73

*Some parameters (pre-diagnostic period, heredity) are based on the personal information given by the patient.
** After 10 years 723 patients were still in the study.

Table 1.3. Diabetic subjects (registered in Bucharest in 1984) without insulin therapy

Parameters	Initial	After 10 years
Total no.: 819 (84.35%)		
Sex: male 412 (50.31%)		
female 407 (46.69%)		
Mean age: 56.68 ± 10.74 years		
Pre-diagnosis period: 19.42 ± 37.32 months		
Diabetes heredity: 14.29%		
BMI	29.25 ± 14.71	28.07 ± 5.16
Glycemia (mg%)	174.30 ± 58.36	179.60 ± 60.57
Glycosuria (g/l)	20.13 ± 16.64	17.22 ± 16.25
Type of treatment (%):		
Diet (only)	38.46	14.28
Sulfonylurea	26.53	40.78
Biguanides	24.30	14.06
Combination	10.74	30.88

(from 38.46% to 14.28%) has been noted as well as a rise (from 26.53% to 40.78%) in those treated with sulfonylurea derivatives, a reduction (from 24.3% to 14.06%) in treatments with biguanides and a noticeable rise (from 10.74% to 30.88%) in patients on combined oral therapy.

Table 1.4 presents essential information on 68 patients who were registered in 1984 as having IDDM or type 1 diabetes. It can be seen that they represent only 7% of the total number of cases registered in that year. From the point of view of insulin therapy, a disappearance of the "conventional" preparations is evident 10 years later (but without an appreciable increase in human insulin) while a significant increase of the mean daily insulin dosage (from 30.25 ± 12.31 IU to 38.95 ± 12.42 IU; $p < 0.01$) is observable.

Table 1.5 presents the principal characteristics of the 81 patients (8.34% of the initial number) to whom insulin therapy was introduced—for various reasons—not at the onset, but later (following an average duration of 5.83 ± 3.64 years). Analysis of this group shows several interesting aspects. If we compare the average age at diagnosis a great difference between IDDM (27–28 years) and "questionable

Table 1.4. Type 1 (insulin-dependent) diabetes patients registered in Bucharest in 1984

Parameters	Initial	After 10 years
Total no.: 68 (7.00%)		
Sex: male 30 (44.12%)		
female 38 (55.88%)		
Mean age: 27.89 ± 17.75 years		
Pre-diagnosis period: 2.80 ± 3.20		
months		
Diabetes heredity: 16.39%		
BMI	21.12 ± 4.29	Data unavailable
Glycemia (mg%)	216.00 ± 140.40	211.00 ± 95.45
Glycosuria (g/l)	29.41 ± 22.65	20.85 ± 15.51
Insulin type (%):		
Coventional	15.39	0
Highly purified	81.33	95.08
Human	3.28	4.92
Insulin dosage (IU/day)	30.25 ± 12.31	38.95 ± 12.42 ($p < 0.01$)

insulin dependency" (about 51 years) can be observed (Figure 1.1). Another very suggestive comparison is that connected with the pre-diagnostic period and the initial body mass index (BMI) (Figure 1.2). The lowest values can be seen with IDDM. In patients with "questionable insulin dependency" these values are much higher but are lower than those associated with NIDDM. It is also interesting to examine insulin dosage (Figure 1.3): I have already mentioned the significant increase seen after 10 years in IDDM patients; the actual insulin dosage for patients with "questionable insulin dependency" is somewhat intermediate.

Long-term follow up has demonstrated that the proportion of patients who could be classified as having "questionable insulin dependency" increases with time and significantly exceeds the number of patients with type 1 diabetes[6]. The clinical profile of this category would be, in general terms, as follows: diabetic subjects who, at the onset, appear to have NIDDM or type 2 diabetes, after several years develop oral drug failure, lose weight, have increasingly

Table 1.5. "Questionable insulin dependency" (patients registered in Bucharest in 1984 and re-evaluated 10 years later)

Parameters	Initial	After 10 years
Total no.: 81 (8.34%)		
Sex: male 38 (46.91%)		
female 43 (53.09%)		
Mean age: 51.54 ± 10.17 years		
Pre-diagnosis period: 13.60 ± 28.48 months		
Diabetes heredity: 14.81%		
Time between registration and insulin treatment: 5.83 ± 3.64		
BMI	25.34 ± 4.50	25.63 ± 3.17
Glycemia (mg%)	214.50 ± 62.81	181.00 ± 56.47 ($p < 0.01$)
Glycosuria (g/l)	23.72 ± 20.16	17.91 ± 19.40 ($p < 0.05$)
Insulin type (%):		
Coventional	–	3.28
Highly purified	–	84.37
Human	–	12.35
Insulin dosage (IU/day)	–	33.47 ± 11.60

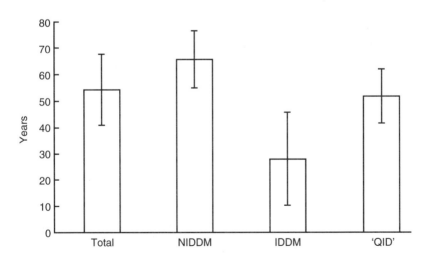

Figure 1.1. Mean age at registration

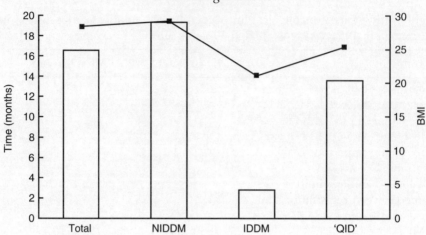

Figure 1.2. Pre-diagnosis period (□) and initial BMI (■)

unsatisfactory metabolic parameters and are obliged to accept insulin therapy which has a salutary effect.

A multicentered study carried out on a large number of first-degree relatives of patients with different types of diabetes mellitus has shown that, in subjects with IDDM, IDDM is predominant amongst their first-degree relatives; in subjects with NIDDM, NIDDM is

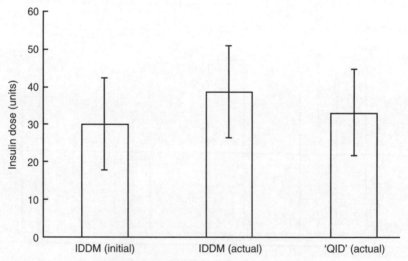

Figure 1.3. Mean insulin dosages

predominant in first-degree relatives (to a greater extent than in the comparable ratio for IDDM) while in subjects with "questionable insulin deficiency" NIDDM—and not "questionable insulin deficiency" or IDDM—is predominant (in a somewhat smaller proportion than with NIDDM subjects). Thus, the connection with inheritance appears to be stronger with NIDDM, even if insulin treatment is the final therapeutic solution for this group of patients[7].

In the terminology proposed for the designation of these patients, aside from "questionable insulin dependency", terms such as "secondary insulin dependency", "intermediate type of diabetes" and "type 2 diabetes with insulin therapy" have also been used. Until the finalizing, dissemination and acceptance of a new classification for the diabetic syndrome, I feel that the term that is most adequate and least open to criticism is that of "insulin-requiring diabetes". This designation has the following advantages for the medical practitioner: it is based on the usual clinical criteria and does not require costly genetic or immunologic tests, it highlights the importance of insulin (without which the patient's state would worsen) and it differentiates this group of patients from those with IDDM and NIDDM.

It is very true, however, that, through the use of in-depth and costly investigations a great proportion of those cases that are difficult to classify may be sorted out. Thus, it has been suggested that basal serum C-peptide, or stimulated C-peptide (following glucose or glucagon stimulation) can be used to discriminate between type 1 and type 2 diabetes. It is likely that a combination of C-peptide and antibodies to glutamic acid decarboxylase will provide even better differentiation[2].

An additional difficulty is, from the point of view of doctrine, the modern tendency to utilize insulin therapy in difficult forms of NIDDM. This trend has a solid clinical and moral justification and is encouraged by most diabetologists even though it is associated with some risk[10,11].

In Figure 1.4, an evaluation of the "gray zone" between IDDM and NIDDM is attempted. In the vicinity of the area occupied by "pure" type 1 diabetes, some subjects who have been erroneously considered as having IDDM may have been included—especially those with "type $1\frac{1}{2}$ diabetes", "slow type 1", "latent IDDM", "latent autoimmune diabetes in adults (LADA)". These terms can be superimposed

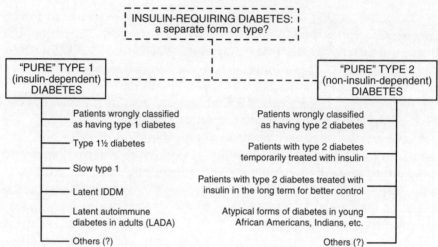

Figure 1.4. Could there be a *terra incognita* between type 1 and type 2 diabetes?

to an extent and lack full scientific support. Close to the area occupied by "pure" type 2 diabetes may be a series of subjects whose classification has been wrongly made; in addition, there are patients with type 2 diabetes who had been treated for a short period with insulin for relatively well defined reasons, patients with type 2 diabetes treated with insulin for long periods for good glycemic control, and young African Americans, Indians or other population groups with atypical diabetes[1,2].

The clinical bases for the eventual consideration of the so-called "insulin-requiring diabetes" as a separate form of diabetes have already been stated.

It remains for us to ask ourselves if the entities mentioned above with more or less well defined characteristics cover the entire area between type 1 and type 2 diabetes mellitus or whether a part of this may still be considered *terra incognita*.

1.3   A NEW CLASSIFICATION IS IN THE OFFING

Suggestions for the improvement of the classification of diabetes mellitus have multiplied considerably[12,13].

An international expert committee on the diagnosis and classification of diabetes mellitus, working under the auspices of the American Diabetes Association (ADA), was established in May 1995 and published a comprehensive report in 1997. This report was divided into four sections: the definition and description of diabetes mellitus; the classification of diabetes mellitus and other categories of glucose regulation; diagnostic criteria for diabetes mellitus; testing for diabetes in presumably healthy individuals[14].

As a consequence of the accumulation of an impressive volume of knowledge related to the causes and mechanisms of the genesis of diabetes, the new classification is a big departure from the older "treatment-based" system and a step in the direction of an etiologic system similar to that which exists for other diseases. The task is incomplete, however, because the precise etiopathogenesis in many cases of type 2 diabetes remains unknown[15].

A shortened form of the proposals advanced by the ADA is given in Table 1.6. The main novelties brought by the new classification are given below.

1. The terms "insulin-dependent diabetes" and "non-insulin-dependent diabetes" which signify the classification of diabetes on the basis of therapy rather than etiology, have been eliminated.
2. The terms "type 1 diabetes" and "type 2 diabetes" (with Arabic numerals) have been maintained. In type 1 diabetes are included cases brought on by a process of beta-cell destruction usually leading to a process of absolute insulin deficiency. These patients are prone to ketoacidosis. The majority of cases result from an autoimmune process but idiopathic forms exist.
3. Most cases fall into the category of type 2 diabetes. The main disorders of these patients may range from predominant insulin resistance with relative insulin deficiency to a predominantly secretory deficit with insulin resistance.
4. The class of "malnutrition-related diabetes mellitus" (MRDM) has been eliminated and fibrocalculus pancreatopathy (formerly a subtype of MRDM) has been reclassified as a disease of the exocrine pancreas.
5. Impaired glucose tolerance (IGT) has been retained and an analogous intermediate stage of fasting glucose designated impaired fasting glucose (IFG).

Preventing Diabetes

Table 1.6. The shortened form of the "etiologic classification of diabetes mellitus" proposed by the American Diabetes Association (1997)

I. Type 1 diabetes* (beta-cell destruction, usually leading to absolute insulin deficiency)
    A. Immune mediated
    B. Idiopathic
II. Type 2 diabetes* (may range from predominant insulin resistance with relative insulin deficiency to a predominantly secretory defect with insulin resistance)
III. Other specific types:
    A. Genetic defects of beta-cell function
    B. Genetic defects in insulin action
    C. Diseases of the exocrine pancreas
    D. Endocrinopathies
    E. Drug—or chemically—induced
    F. Infections
    G. Uncommon forms of immune-mediated diabetes
    H. Other genetic syndromes sometimes associated with diabetes
IV. Gestational diabetes mellitus (GDM)

---

*Patients with any form of diabetes may require insulin treatment at some stage of their disease. Such use of insulin does not, of itself, classify the patient. Adapted from reference 14

6. The term "gestational diabetes mellitus" (GDM) has been retained.
7. The degree of hyperglycemia (if any) may change with time, reflecting the extent of the underlying disease process. The severity of the metabolic disturbance increases, diminishes or remains the same.
8. Many diabetic subjects do not easily fit into a single class. For the clinician, it is less important to label the particular type of diabetes than it is to understand the pathogenesis of the hyperglycemia and to treat it effectively[14].

It is to be expected that additional information will accumulate and clarification of the new recommendations will inevitably occur. At present, however, the ADA and other important scientific authorities strongly recommend that the new classification and diagnostic criteria be adopted, promulgated and implemented[15].

A WHO consultation has taken place in parallel with the report of the ADA Expert Committee to re-examine diagnostic criteria and classification. In general, similar conclusions were reached[5]. In the provisional report of the WHO consultation, the classification defines both process and stage of the disease. The processes include the type 1 autoimmune and non-autoimmune, with beta-cell destruction; type 2 with varying degrees of insulin resistance and insulin hyposecretion; GDM and "other types" where the cause is known (e.g. MODY, endocrinopathies). It is anticipated that this group will expand as causes of type 2 become known. Stages range from normoglycemia to insulin required for survival. It is hoped that the new classification will allow better categorization of individuals and lead to fewer therapeutic misjudgements[5].

Discussions about the proposals and suggestions related to the classification of diabetes mellitus continue[16–21], but there are clear intentions to form the most significant observations and comments and to forward the proposals to WHO for approval[5].

REFERENCES

1. Bennett PH. Definition, Diagnosis and Classification of Diabetes Mellitus and Impaired Glucose Tolerance. In Kahn CR, Weir GC (eds). *Joslin's Diabetes Mellitus*, 13th edn. Philadelphia: Lea & Febiger, 1994; 193–200.
2. Harris MI, Zimmet P. Classification of Diabetes Mellitus and Other Categories of Glucose Intolerance. In Alberti KGMM, Zimmet P, DeFronzo RA, Keen H (eds). *International Textbook of Diabetes Mellitus*, 2nd edn. Chichester: Wiley, 1997; 9–23.
3. WHO Expert Committee on Diabetes Mellitus. *Second Report*. Geneva: World Health Organization, 1980.
4. *WHO Diabetes Mellitus. Report of a WHO Study Group*. Geneva: World Health Organization, 1985.
5. Alberti KGGM, Zimmet PZ for the WHO Consultation. Definition, Diagnosis and Classification of Diabetes Mellitus and its Complications. Part 1: Diagnosis and Classification of Diabetes Mellitus. Provisional Report of a WHO Consultation. *Diabetic Med* 1998; **15**: 539–553.
6. Mincu I, Ionescu-Tirgoviste C, Dumitrescu C, Cheta D, Popa E, Strachinariu R. Secondary insulin dependence: type 1 or type 2 diabetes? *Diabetes Res Clin Pract* 1985; suppl. 1: S381.

7. Cheţa D, Dumitrescu C, Georgescu M *et al.* A study on the types of diabetes mellitus in first degree relatives of diabetic patients. *Diabete Metab* 1990; **16**: 11–15.
8. Tuomi T, Groop LD, Zimmet PZ, Rowley MJ, Knowles W, Mackay IR. Antibodies to glutamic acid decarboxylase reveal latent autoimmune diabetes mellitus in adults with a non-insulin-dependent onset of disease. *Diabetes* 1993; **42**: 359–362.
9. Hagopian WA, Karlsen AE, Gottsater A *et al.* Quantitative assay using recombinant human islet glutamic acid decarboxylase (GAD 65) shows that 64K autoantibody positivity at onset predicts diabetes type. *J Clin Invest* 1993; **91**: 368–374.
10. Rosenzweig JL. Principles of Insulin Therapy. In Kahn CR, Weir GC (eds). *Joslin's Diabetes Mellitus*, 13th edn. Philadelphia: Lea & Febiger, 1994; 460–488.
11. Peters AL, Davidson MB. Aging and Diabetes. In Alberti KGMM, Zimmet P, DeFronzo RA, Keen H (eds). *International Textbook of Diabetes Mellitus*, 2nd edn. Chichester: Wiley, 1997; 1151–1176.
12. Service FJ, Rizza RA, Zimmermann BR, Dyck PJ, O'Brien PC, Melton III LJ. The classification of diabetes by clinical and C-peptide criteria. A prospective population-based study. *Diabetes Care* 1997; **20**: 198–201.
13. Kuzuya T, Matsuda A. Classification of diabetes on the basis of etiologies versus degree of insulin deficiency. *Diabetes Care* 1997; **20**: 219–220.
14. Report of the Expert Committee on the Diagnosis and Classification of Diabetes Mellitus. *Diabetes Care* 1997; **20**: 1183–1197.
15. Eastman RC, Vincor F. Science: Moving us in the right direction. *Diabetes Care* 1997; **20**: 1057–1058.
16. Guillausseau PJ. Classification et critères diagnostiques du diabète: propositions de l'ADA et de l'OMS. *Diabete Metab* 1997; **23**: 454–455.
17. Fajans SS. Revised etiologic classification of diabetes (letter). *Diabetes Care* 1998; **21**: 466–467.
18. Sims EA, Catalano PM. Response to the Expert Committee on the Diagnosis and Classification of Diabetes Mellitus (letter). *Diabetes Care* 1998; **21**: 467–468.
19. Service FJ. New classification of diabetes (letter). *Diabetes Care* 1998; **21**: 469–470.
20. Zarbock SF. New recommendations to diagnose and classify diabetes: important implications for home care. *Home Care Provider* 1998; **3**: 77–78.
21. Zimmet P, Alberti G, deCourten MP. New classification and criteria for diabetes: moving the goalposts closer (editorial). *Med J Aust* 1998; **168**: 593–594.

2

Overview of the Etiopathogenesis of Type 1 Diabetes

The knowledge on the etiopathogenesis of type 1 diabetes mellitus has increased greatly in recent years, influencing the clinical, therapeutic and even prophylactic aspects of this disorder[1]. This chapter is not intended to be an exhaustive presentation of the problem but only a synthesis of the principal causes and mechanisms involved, which also have a close connection with the means of prediction and prevention.

2.1 ETIOLOGIC FACTORS AND PATHOGENIC MECHANISMS OF TYPE 1 DIABETES MELLITUS

The following will be touched upon only briefly: genetic basis, environmental factors, pathogenic autoimmune concept, therapeutic consequences and some insufficiently clarified aspects.

2.1.1 Genetic Basis

It has been known for a long time that type 1 diabetes is a familial disorder. About 1 in 20 first-degree relatives of individuals with type 1 diabetes will develop the disease (compared with 4 in 1000 in the general population)[2,3]. A prospective study of identical twins from the UK yielded a concordance of approximately 36%, and is probably the most accurate estimate available[4].

The genetic background of different autoimmune diseases was more firmly established by human leukocyte antigen (HLA) typing, which demonstrated that some HLA alleles occur in higher frequencies in subjects with certain diseases than in the general population. Analysis of type 1 diabetes shows both positive and negative associations with HLA alleles: HLA-DR3 or HLA-DR4 was observed in 90–95% of Caucasians with this disorder but in only 40% of normal subjects; nearly 50% of type 1 diabetics are HLA-DR3/DR4 heterozygotes (in contrast with 5% of normal individuals). The HLA-DQ alleles are even more strongly associated with type 1 diabetics than the DR alleles[3]. With the availability of neucleotide sequences, each polymorphic allele is assigned a number for its DQA and DQB chain[2]. As Nepom emphasized, the highest genetic risk attributed to the HLA complex is in subjects who are heterogeneous at the HLA-DQB1 locus and carry both a *0302 and a *0201 allele. These individuals are more than 15 times as likely to get type 1 diabetes before the age of 30 as those who do not have such a genotype[5]. On the other hand, some HLA haplotypes confer protection from the disease. For instance, haplotypes bearing DR2 alleles usually protect from diabetes independently of whether the other HLA haplotype contains a high-risk allele[3]. A "dominant protection" is ensured by a specific HLA haplotype that is positive for DQB1*0602[5].

The evidence for susceptibility to at least two forms of type 1 diabetes comes from the observations, made during familial aggregation studies, that DR3 susceptibility acts in a recessive fashion and that DR4-related susceptibility seems to act in a dominant fashion. A phenotypic heterogeneity is also apparent between HLA-DR3 and DR4-associated diabetes. The DR3 (autoimmune) form is characterized by a higher persistence of islet cell antibodies and antipancreatic cell-mediated immunity but a relative lack of antibodies to exogenous insulin. The DR4 form is accompanied by an increased response to exogenous insulin, appears to have an earlier age of onset, presents seasonally and may be related to viral infections[6].

The proportion of genetic susceptibility to type 1 diabetes accounted for by the HLA region is in the range of 60–70%. Other non-HLA loci play a role in type 1 diabetes. Over the past 20 years, a number of non-MHC candidate genes have been studied and as many as ten loci have now been identified by mapping in humans[1,6,7]. The best studied markers include the loci for tumor necrosis factor (TNF), heat shock protein 70 (hsp 70), TAP/LMP and C4[7]. A summary of human type 1 diabetes loci is presented in Table 2.1.

Thus, the strong genetic associations of type 1 diabetes with HLA genes renders certain HLA alleles good markers of disease risk. Modern DNA techniques have enabled rapid increase in our knowledge of these genes and of their associations with type 1 diabetes. However, there has been little progress in mapping susceptibility to the disease more precisely within the major histocompatibility complex (MHC). Special attention has focused on the role of DQβ–Asp57 and specific heterodimers in disease susceptibility but these could not adequately explain the observed HLA associations in different populations[8].

In the future, the identification of genetic susceptibility markers will lead to the isolation of individual genes and their responsible polymorphisms. The pathophysiology of type 1 diabetes will thus be better understood and new therapeutic and preventive strategies will be developed[1,8].

2.1.2 Environmental Factors

The possibility that some viruses and toxic substances are involved in the production of type 1 diabetes has been under discussion for a long

Table 2.1. Summary of genetic loci of human type 1 diabetes

Locus	Chromosome
IDDM 1 (HLA)	6p
IDDM 2 (5' insulin gene VNTR)	11p
IDDM 3	15q
IDDM 4	11q
IDDM 5	6q
IDDM 7	2q
Others	3q,4q,6q,13q

Adapted from reference 6

time. The importance of environmental factors in type 1 diabetes is clearly indicated by the concordance rate in identical twins (mentioned earlier), by the geographic differences in the incidence of the disease and by the increasing incidence during the past few decades[9]. But the list of environmental factors and information about them has increased considerably in recent years and essential contributions in this direction have been made by large projects evaluating the epidemiology of diabetes in children and adolescents (DIAMOND, EURODIAB, etc.)[10,11].

2.1.2.1 Viruses

The hypothesis of the involvement of viruses in diabetogenesis is being heatedly debated and is based on the following arguments: its abrupt clinical onset, the seasonal variation of the disease, the presence of inflammatory cells in the islets (insulitis) and destruction of beta cells, the temporal relationship between viral infections (mumps, rubella, Coxsackie B group) and the appearance of diabetes, epidemiologic research demonstrating a correlation between raised antibody titers of specific antiviral antibodies (e.g. for Coxsackie B group of viruses) and the increased frequency of type 1 diabetes as well as the existence of some animal models of diabetes induced with the aid of viruses[1].

More recently, molecular techniques have been used to determine the prevalence of viral DNA. Human cytomegalovirus (CMV) genes were discovered in 22% of type 1 diabetics (compared with 2.6% of controls)[12]. It has been suggested that persistent CMV infection may be relevant to pathogenesis in some cases of type 1 diabetes[6]. It is interesting to note that elimination of natural mumps infection in Finland (by vaccination) has decreased the incidence of type 1 diabetes in that nation[13]. Measles vaccination also correlates with a lower risk of disease[14].

The contribution of a viral component to the etiology of diabetes is strongly supported by animal studies. These suggest that an infectious agent can induce diabetes in at least four different ways:

- Acute infection of the islet beta cells leading to necrosis: encephalomyocarditis (EMC) virus and reoviruses
- Autoimmune mechanisms: rubella and Kilham's rat virus (KRV)

- Persistent infection leading to decreased growth and lifespan of the islet beta cells: lymphocytic choriomeningitis virus (LCMV)
- Biochemical disturbances of the cell or cell membrane, leading to decreased insulin synthesis release: Venezuelan encephalitis virus[6,15].

It is felt that viruses may be involved in the pathogenesis of human type 1 diabetes, in at least two distinct ways. Firstly, viruses may directly infect and destroy the beta cells, resulting in clinical disease. Alternatively, since a lot of cases are known to involve a rather long diabetogenic process, it is also possible that viruses may trigger or contribute to the autoimmune destruction of the insulin-producing cells[16]. It is also thought that the best human models of infectious agents in type 1 diabetes come from studies with the congenital rubella syndrome and from serial studies of children with viral infections who subsequently developed diabetes[6].

There has been a recent resurgence of reports that type 1 diabetes may be associated with enteroviral infections[17]. The Diabetes Auto-immunity Study in the Young (DAISY) is focusing on potential interactions between HLA class II genes and enteroviral infections[18]. Future studies will examine interactions between viral infections and non-HLA candidate genes[17].

However, the connection between viruses and diabetes appears to be more complicated than could be seen a few years ago. The appearance of the spontaneous animal models of diabetes (BB rats and NOD mice), raised under virus-free conditions, has brought about a change in opinion on the role of viruses in type 1 diabetes. Nowadays it is thought that there are two diabetogenic groups of viruses: some of which induce or hasten the onset of diabetes and others which suppress or prevent its development[3,19]. At this point, interesting speculations have been raised in relation to the possibility of preventive action of some viruses in human type 1 diabetes and on the mechanism of this effect[16].

2.1.2.2   Chemical Agents and Toxins

A number of chemicals have been used to produce diabetes. These substances could be divided into two categories:

(1) with irreversible action—e.g. streptozotocin, alloxan, zinc chelating compounds, pentamidine, pyriminil;
(2) with reversible action—e.g. 6-aminonicotinamide, L-asparaginase, azide, cyanide, cyproheptadine, dehydroascorbic acid, fluoride, iodoacetate, malonate, thiazide, 2-deoxyglucose, manoheptulose[1,20].

Alloxan and a single large dose of streptozotocin may act at several sites in the beta cell such as the glucose transport mechanism at the level of the cell membrane, the sulphydryl groups of glucokinase and at the mitochondria by inducing the formation of free radicals or by inducing DNA strand breaks[21]. Such DNA alteration stimulates DNA repair by the nuclear poly(ADP-ribose) synthetase and brings about a depletion of cellular NAD[22]. Not all authors confirm this similarity of action between alloxan and streptozotocin[19].

In contrast, it has been demonstrated that repeated injections of low doses of streptozotocin into susceptible mice can induce a form of diabetes similar to human type 1, in which the participation of cell-mediated immunity and the coexistence of a marked pancreatic insulitis are encountered[23]. However, this form of diabetes should be differentiated from the autoimmune type seen in the spontaneous animal models[19]. Recently, it has been shown that apoptosis is the mode of cell death responsible for beta cell loss in the multiple low-dose streptozotocin model of type 1 diabetes[24].

Vacor (pyriminil) is a nitrosourea derivative used as a rodenticide. It is able to produce an insulin-dependent diabetes including ketoacidosis, which is a result of beta cell destruction[25]. The course of the diabetogenic process is similar to that observed for streptozotocin. Dietary nitrosamines (present in some smoked meats) can determine beta cell alteration and diabetes[21]. Zinc chelating compounds (such as dithizone and 8-hydroxyquinolone) are also known to bring about permanent diabetes in rabbits and mice[26]. Pentamidine, proposed for the therapy of pneumonia produced by *Pneumocystis carinii* could produce hypoglycemia followed occasionally by diabetes[1,20].

2.1.2.3 Nutritional Factors

Food additives (*N*-nitroso compounds) have already been mentioned. Coffee and sugar have been included on the list of potential triggers of diabetes, starting from the moderate correlation between the per capita consumption of these nutrients and national diabetes incidence rates[27].

Several epidemiological and ecological studies have suggested that the early utilization of cows' milk protein in the nourishment of infants could be a factor for the induction of the autoimmune process leading to type 1 diabetes[9,27]. The accumulated evidence provided the basis for the recommendation by the American Academy of Pediatrics to avoid cows' milk introduction in infants at risk for the development of type 1 diabetes[28]. Other studies have not confirmed this association[29]; furthermore, preliminary findings of the DAISY study suggest a protective effect of early cows' milk feeding[30].

Initial studies have focused on bovine serum albumin (BSA). Antibodies to this component were discovered in sera from most type 1 diabetic individuals as well as in BB rats and NOD mice. These antibodies were directed against a 17-amino acid peptide (ABBOS) of BSA and precipitated a 64 kDa protein from islet cell lysates. T-cell reactivity was also demonstrated against the ABBOS fragment and the islet cell protein[9]. Interest has concentrated also on β lactoglobulin (BLG). Antibodies to BLG were reported as independent risk factors for type 1 diabetes and enhanced cellular immune response to BLG was noticed in individuals with recent-onset disease[31]. Casein is the major protein in cows' milk and comprises four fractions (alpha, beta, gamma and kappa). The beta casein seems to be the most likely candidate antigen as antibodies to bovine beta casein and T lymphocytes recognizing it are detectable in most type 1 diabetes patients at diagnosis[32].

The identification of a compound in cows' milk able to induce the activation of autoreactive T lymphocytes may be important for the understanding of the pathogenesis of type 1 diabetes and the possibility of preventing the disease. In fact, the protein content of infant milk formulae is an easily modifiable factor for the prevention of type 1 diabetes[9].

2.1.2.4   Other Factors

The risk of the appearance of type 1 diabetes depends on the average annual temperature, distance from the equator, ethnic characteristics of the population, type of cutaneous pigmentation and reactivity to ultraviolet light. The remarkable differences between the north and south have provoked many comments. For instance, a child born in Finland has a 10 times greater risk of developing diabetes than one born in northern Greece[11].

2.1.3 The Concept of the Autoimmune Pathogenesis

Most authors consider type 1 diabetes to be an autoimmune disease although doctrinal criteria for such a characterization are not totally satisfied.

2.1.3.1 *Autoantigens*

At least two of the specific antigens of so-called islet cell antibodies (ICAs) have been identified as insulin and glutamic acid decarboxylase (GAD). The continuing search for other antigens has led to the discovery of numerous islet cell components to which antibodies in the sera of new diabetic patients bind[33]. Some of them are non-protein antigens (lipids or glycolipids); for instance, an islet sialoglycolipid and sulphatides. Of the long list of protein antigens, here are the principal examples: GLUT-2 (beta cell glucose transporter), chymotrypsinogen, carboxypeptidase H, heat shock proteins, ABBOS (mentioned above)[1,33,34]. The problem of autoantigens in type 1 diabetes remains open. There is promise of antigen-specific immune intervention therapies to prevent diabetes in those identified as being at risk[35].

2.1.3.2 *Autoantibodies*

Although in the sera of many diabetics many circulating antibodies have been identified, not one of them can be considered as being of primary importance—rather they are the consequences of a polymorphic and polyclonal activation of B lymphocytes—some of them may none the less serve as valuable markers of the process of beta-cell destruction[34].

Cytoplasmic ICAs. These were first reported in 1974 and have been the most widely studied to date. After prolonged discussions, their evaluation is now standardized in the Juvenile Diabetes Foundation (JDF) units. This family of IgG antibodies recognizes more islet components with ganglioside characteristics. The presence of ICAs has been demonstrated in 60–80% of newly diagnosed type 1 diabetics, in about 3% of first-degree relatives of type 1 diabetics and in 0.2% of the general population[36]. The prevalence and titer of ICAs fall in relation to the duration of the disease. The high titer of ICAs predicts a rapid loss of beta-cell function following diagnosis. Their presence, especially in high titers, increases the risk of the appearance of type 1 diabetes in the families of patients and even in the general population. It could be said that, at present, ICAs constitute an important scientific instrument for the prediction of type 1 diabetes[37].

Insulin autoantibodies (IAA). These represent another immunologic marker for the detection of subjects at risk for type 1 diabetes. They are present in about 60% of newly discovered type 1 diabetics before insulin therapy and show an inverse correlation with age. The IAA concentration seems to be closely related to the rate of autoimmune beta-cell destruction[36]. IAA have also been found in insulin autoimmune syndrome, thyroid disease, systemic lupus erythematosus and rheumatoid arthritis[38].

Antibodies to GAD. The first successful attempts at distinguishing islet components recognized by autoantibodies in type 1 diabetes were published in 1982 and were referred to as the "64k-antigen"[39,40]. In 1990, the 64k-antigen was identified as the enzyme glutamic acid decarboxylase. It is evident now that GAD antibodies occupy an important position in the immune pathogenesis of type 1 diabetes and also the stiff-man syndrome. Dissection of the GAD antibody response may uncover antibody subspecificities recognizing specific epitopes on GAD that are more closely associated with type 1 diabetes and that can be useful for its prediction[40].

Other autoantibodies. A variety of autoantibodies can be observed in the sera of patients with type 1 diabetes, particularly at the beginning of the clinical disease. Besides the three forms already presented, it is thought that antibodies to the 37 kDa and 40 kDa autoantigen (ICA 512/IA-2 and IA-2β) have enough diabetes specificity to be used as markers of risk in first-degree relatives[36].

2.1.3.3   *Cellular Immunity*

Despite the usefulness of autoantibodies as markers for the disease, there is much data that suggests that type 1 diabetes results from cell-mediated destruction of islet beta cells. Amongst these are: (a) the demonstration of beta-cell antigen-specific T-cell responses in type 1 diabetics and in individuals at increased risk for the disease; (b) the mononuclear infiltrate of the pancreatic islets; (c) observations of animal models which show that T cells are required for and actively involved in beta-cell damage (adoptive transfer, lymphocyte depletion, etc.); (d) the encouraging response of human subjects with type 1 diabetes to immunospecific therapy aimed at cellular immunity. Based on these arguments, it is thought that markers of cellular immunity will prove superior to antibody markers in terms of their ability to delineate the natural history of type 1 diabetes as well as to determine the individual risk for the disease[41].

2.1.3.4   *Insulitis*

The characteristic lesion in the pancreas of type 1 diabetics is an infiltrate of lymphocytes in the islets, sometimes accompanied by macrophages and neutrophils[3]. Most infiltrating lymphocytes discovered in the islets of a patient who died at diagnosis were CD8[+] T cells[42]. The term *insulitis* has been used for these changes. The more chronic the disease becomes, the more the beta cells of the islets are progressively depleted and, in many cases with a prolonged course, are no longer discernible. During the initial phases of insulitis, there appears to be increased expression of class I MHC molecules by the cells comprising the islets of Langerhans. In addition to enhanced expression of class I MHC, there is evidence that the beta cells may also be expressing class II MHC molecules[3,42,43].

The final destruction of beta cells is probably the result of many factors as it is dependent on multiple cell types (macrophages, CD4[+] and CD8[+] lymphocytes) and multiple mechanisms (free radical damage, cytokines, CD8[+] T-cell-mediated toxicity)[2,3].

2.1.3.5   *Course of the Autoimmune Process*

Progression to overt type 1 diabetes can be divided into more stages, starting with genetic susceptibility[36,44]. A precipitating event (either mutational or environmental) presumably triggers the autoimmune attack against the pancreatic beta cells. The presence at this stage of antibodies directed against islet cell-related antigens can be used for the identification of subjects at high risk of developing the disease. With the continuation of the islet destructive activity, in addition to the immune abnormality, individuals present a progressive loss of first-phase insulin release. They are still normoglycemic. Modified insulin secretion is one of the first metabolic changes during the "preclinical" phase of the disease. In the 18 months before the clinical onset of diabetes, a subclinical rise of glycemia is often detected[45]. The loss of first-phase insulin release is followed by hyperglycemia and the clinical onset of the disease. C-peptide production can continue for a period but ends once the autoimmune process completely destroys the islet beta cells[36].

2.1.4 Therapeutic Consequences

The autoimmune pathogenic concept constitutes a solid scientific basis for the treatment of type 1 diabetes mellitus. The substitutive character of insulin therapy and its absolute necessity (the insulin-dependence of these patients) become clearly evident and are a decisive element for the constitution of specific education programs, without which proper care is not possible.

On the other hand, the chief outlines of immunotherapeutic methods for type 1 diabetes mellitus should be drawn. Necessary to the success of this is the existence of beta-cell secretory activity sufficient to permit the restoration of normal glucose metabolism once the destructive autoimmune process had been suppressed[2].

2.1.5 Insufficiently Clarified Aspects

With all the progress made in recent years, the etiopathogenicity of type 1 diabetes mellitus still presents unclear aspects which make prediction and prevention more difficult.

The genetics of this disease remain an area of some confusion. There is no consensus as to which gene(s) or combination of genes in the

MHC is responsible for the HLA-related susceptibility or how many other genes outside of the HLA region (in most cases on other chromosomes) are involved. The analysis of the genetics of type 1 diabetes is beset with some major difficulties. Among these are: (a) the reduced penetrance of the disorder; (b) the confounding of linkage and association; (c) the heterogeneity within the disorder itself[6].

The possibility that environmental agents have a significant contribution to the etiopathogenesis of type 1 diabetes mellitus must be thoroughly investigated, especially with regard to the implications for preventive strategies. Environmental factors could play one of several different roles[5,46]. They might function as initiating events—i.e. events which begin or continue the etiologic processes. If environmental factors have this role then more than one might be involved. In contrast, environmental agents could act mainly as precipitating factors (that is, factors which convert preclinical diabetes into clinical disease)[6]. Unfortunately, the list of environmental factors is incomplete and the contributions already discussed not absolutely certain.

The relative importance of genetic and environmental factors in the causation of type 1 diabetes is unknown. Muntoni *et al.* studied this question by assessing the incidence of the disease in children born in a region with a low incidence of type 1 diabetes (Lazio), but whose parents come from a region with high incidence (Sardinia). The results show that two different ethnic groups living in the same region have a fourfold difference in incidence of type 1 diabetes. Children of Sardinian heritage born in Lazio have the same incidence as that in the population of origin, which is genetically prone to the disease. Moreover, children with one Sardinian parent had a rate half that of Sardinians and double that of the indigenous population. The authors concluded that, in a given population, genetic susceptibility determines the frequency of type 1 diabetes in response to the environmental challenge[47].

The autoimmune pathogenic theory has not been 100% proven. As has already been mentioned the islet autoantigen(s) is(are) not yet precisely identified. Another significant objection that can be made about this theory is the lack of proof that the serum from lymphocytes of human patients maintain the capacity to transfer the disease[1].

Finally, there are type 1 diabetics in whom no evidence of autoimmunity is present. According to the Expert Committee of the ADA, these cases might be classified as idiopathic type[48].

2.2   PREDICTION AND PREVENTION OF TYPE 1 DIABETES MELLITUS FROM ITS ETIOPATHOGENESIS

In Table 2.2 a summary of the etiology and pathogenesis of type 1 diabetes mellitus in connection with the material above is presented. The suggestions and practical aspects related to the prediction and prevention of the disease are derived, in essence, on the most demonstrated data of this complex problem.

2.2.1   General Aspects of the Prediction of Type 1 Diabetes Mellitus

Identification of the individuals at risk of type 1 diabetes mellitus is of great importance since an intervention during the prodromal phase is

Table 2.2. Factors and mechanisms involved in the causation of type 1 diabetes mellitus (general view)

Genetic susceptibility (background):
- MHC genes
- Non-MHC genes

Environmental factors (triggers):
- Viruses
- Chemicals and drugs
- Nutritional factors
- Others

Autoimmune process (pathogenesis):
- Autoantigens
- Autoantibodies
- Cellular immunity
- Effector mechanisms
- Insulitis
- Progressive deterioration of insulin secretion

Main clinical consequences:
- Type 1 diabetes is an autoimmune disorder
- Insulin dependency

the most likely means of preventing subsequent morbidity and mortality[36]. Predictive methods are proposed especially in the following circumstances:

- To prevent morbidity at onset (taking into consideration that 1 in 200 children die at the onset of diabetes)
- To aid in family and career decisions
- To screen first-degree relatives for entry into preventive trials
- Subjects with history of transient hyperglycemia
- To avoid diabetes in potential renal transplant donors
- To aid in the diagnosis of type 1 versus type 2 diabetes[2,36]

The prediction of type 1 diabetes is based, generally speaking, on genetic markers, humoral immune markers, T-cell markers and metabolic assessment in the preclinical period. A comprehensive documentation of this is contained in the work *Prediction, Prevention and Genetic Counseling in IDDM*[49].

According to Hahl *et al.*, the strategy for predicting type 1 diabetes may be concentrated on: (1) repeated analyses of marker(s) of disease-associated autoimmunity in the entire population (the pure immunology strategy) or (2) initial evaluation of genetic diabetes susceptibility, followed by repeated measurement of the autoimmune markers only in the smaller, susceptibility restricted individuals (the genetically targeted strategy). The investigations and calculations made by the authors demonstrate that the genetically targeted prediction strategy is remarkably cost-saving compared with the pure immune strategy mainly because fewer subjects will need retesting during follow up[50].

According to Eisenbarth *et al.*, a dual-parameter model (involving two variables; first-phase insulin secretion and levels of IAAs) aids in the prediction of time to diabetes among ICA-positive relatives[51]. The Islet Cell Antibody Register Users Study (ICARUS) register included 456 first-degree relatives with ICA levels ≥ 5 JDF units confirmed in a reference laboratory, 108 of whom progressed to type 1 diabetes in the course of prospective follow up. Analysis of this data set confirmed the importance of the loss of first-phase insulin response, high ICA titer, coexistence of IAA and young age in enhancing the risk of progression to the disease[52].

The major disadvantage of prediction procedures in type 1 diabetes appears to be psychological stress. It is thought that extending these to the general population is still infeasible[36].

2.2.2 General Aspects of the Prevention of Type 1 Diabetes Mellitus

The prevention of type 1 diabetes mellitus has a strong experimental basis, especially with regard to studies carried out in NOD mice and BB rats. The great importance of these studies has prompted us to give them a separate chapter (Chapter 3). In general, it can be said that preventive methods originating from all the factors and all the stages of the etiopathogenesis of this disease have been tried. Thus, for example, the possibilities for the prevention of type 1 diabetes directed at genomic modification or influencing environmental agents have been evaluated. A long list of methods includes immunosuppression, immunotherapy, immunomodulation and tolerance induction as well as the protection of the beta cell from autoimmune attack[19,36].

Prevention of the human type of diabetes mellitus can be implemented by either a high-risk or a population-based approach. The high-risk approach includes identification of susceptible individuals (e.g. first- and second-degree relatives of the patients), and prevention of onset of the disease by modifying the genetic background or precipitating environmental factors. The population-based approach would be more difficult and would aim either at altering lifestyles or at eliminating environmental components that are known to be risk factors for type 1 diabetes[53,54].

Transference (or attempts at transference) of the encouraging results obtained in experimental diabetes have been made. However, it is not expected that primary prevention of type 1 diabetes will be fully possible in the near future because some key points (environmental factors especially) are still missing from our knowledge of the pathogenesis of diabetes[55].

REFERENCES

1. Cheța D. Pathogenesis of Childhood and Adolescent Diabetes. In Șerban V, Brink S (eds). *Childhood and Adolescent Diabetes Mellitus*. Timișoara: Editura de Vest, 1996; 33–50.
2. Eisenbarth GS, Ziegler AD, Colman PA. Pathogenesis of Insulin-dependent (Type I) Diabetes Mellitus. In Kahn CR, Weir GC (eds). *Joslin's Diabetes Mellitus*, 13th edn. Philadelphia: Lea & Febiger, 1994; 216–239.

3. Mehta V, Palmer JP. The Natural History of the IDDM Disease Process. In Palmer JP (ed.). *Prediction, Prevention and Genetic Counseling in IDDM*. Chichester: Wiley, 1996; 3–16.
4. Olmos P, Hern RA, Heaton DA *et al*. The significance of the concordance rate for type 1 (insulin-dependent) diabetes in identical twins. *Diabetologia* 1988; **31**: 747–750.
5. Nepom GT. Genetic Markers in IDDM: the MHC. In Palmer JP (ed.). *Prediction, Prevention and Genetic Counseling in IDDM*. Chichester: Wiley, 1996; 19–26.
6. Scheuner MT, Raffel LJ, Rotter JI. Genetics of Diabetes. In Alberti KGMM, Zimmet P, DeFronzo RA, Keen H (eds). *International Textbook of Diabetes Mellitus*, 2nd edn. Chichester: Wiley, 1977; 37–88.
7. Pociot F, Nerup J. Genetic Markers in IDDM: non-MHC. In Palmer JP (ed.). *Prediction, Prevention and Genetic Counseling in IDDM*. Chichester: Wiley, 1996; 27–42.
8. Cavan DA, Penny MA, Bain SC, Barnett AH. Molecular Genetics of Type 1 Diabetes Mellitus. In Alberti KGMM, Zimmet P, DeFronzo RA, Keen H (eds). *International Textbook of Diabetes Mellitus*, 2nd edn. Chichester: Wiley, 1997; 109–124.
9. Pozilli P. Cow's milk and type 1 diabetes: new evidence about β casein. *Pract Diabet Intern* 1998; **15**: 49–50.
10. Karvonen M, Tuomilheto J, Libman I, Laporte R. A review of the recent epidemiologic data on the worldwide incidence of type 1 (insulin-dependent) diabetes mellitus. World Health Organisation DIAMOND Project Group. *Diabetologia* 1993; **36**: 883–892.
11. Green A, Gale EA, Patterson CC. Incidence of childhood-onset insulin-dependent diabetes mellitus: the EURODIAB ACE Study. *Lancet* 1992; **339**: 905–909.
12. Pak CY, Eun HM, McArthur RG, Yoon JW. Association of cytomegalovirus infection with autoimmune type 1 diabetes. *Lancet* 1988; **ii**: 1–4.
13. Hyöty H, Hiltumen M, Reunanen A *et al*. Decline of mumps antibodies in type 1 (insulin-dependent) diabetic children and a plateau in the rising incidence of type 1 diabetes after introduction of the mumps measles-rubella vaccine in Finland. Childhood Diabetes in Finland Study Group. *Diabetologia* 1993; **36**: 1303–1308.
14. Blom L, Nystrom L, Dahlquist G. The Swedish Childhood Diabetes Study. Vaccinations and infections as risk determinants for diabetes in childhood. *Diabetologia* 1991; **334**: 176–181.
15. Yoon JM. Induction and prevention of type 1 diabetes mellitus by viruses. *Diabete Metab* 1992; **18**: 378–386.
16. Yoon JM. Environmental Factors: Viruses. In Palmer JP (ed.). *Prediction,*

Prevention and Genetic Counseling in IDDM. Chichester: Wiley, 1996; 145–165.
17. Graves PM, Norris JM, Pallansch MA, Gerling IC, Revers M. The role of enteroviral infections in the development of IDDM. Limitations and current approaches. *Diabetes* 1997; **46**: 161–168.
18. Rewers M, Bugawan TL, Norris JM *et al.* Newborn screening for HLA markers associated with IDDM: Diabetes Autoimmunity Study in the Young (DAISY). *Diabetologia* 1996; **39**: 807–812.
19. Cheţa D. Animal models of type 1 (insulin-dependent) diabetes mellitus. *J Pediatr Endocrinol Metab* 1998; **11**: 11–19.
20. Mordes JP, Rossini AA. Animal models of diabetes. *Am J Med* 1981; **70**: 353–360.
21. Bone AJ, Gwillian DJ. Animal models of insulin-dependent diabetes mellitus. In Pickup JC, Williams G (eds). *Textbook of Diabetes*, vol. 16, 2nd edn. Oxford: Blackwell Science, 1997; 1–16.
22. Yamamoto H, Uchigata Y, Okamoto H. Streptozotocin and alloxan induce DNA strand breaks and poly (ADP-ribose) synthetase in pancreatic islets. *Nature* 1981; **103**: 1014–1020.
23. Like AA, Rossini AA. Streptozotocin-induced pancreatic insulitis: a new model of diabetes mellitus. *Science* 1976; **193**: 415–417.
24. O'Brein BA, Harmon BV, Cameron DP, Allan DJ. Beta-cell apoptosis is responsible for the development of IDDM in the multiple low-dose-streptozotocin model. *J Pathol* 1996; **178**: 176–181.
25. LeWitt PA. The neurotoxicity of the rat poison vacor: a clinical study of 12 cases. *N Engl J Med* 1980; **302**: 73–77.
26. Kadota I. Studies on experimental diabetes produced by organic reagents. *J Lab Clin Med* 1950; **35**: 568–591.
27. Karges WJP, Dosch H-M. Environmental Factors: Milk and Others. In Palmer JP (ed.). *Prediction, Prevention and Genetic Counseling in IDDM*. Chichester: Wiley, 1996; 167–180.
28. American Academy of Pediatrics, Work Group on Cow's Milk Proteins and Diabetes. Infant feeding practices and their possible relationship to the etiology of diabetes mellitus. *Pediatrics* 1994; **94**: 752–754.
29. Bodington MJ, McNally PG, Burden AC. Cow's milk and type 1 childhood diabetes–no increase in risk. *Diabetes Med* 1994; **11**: 663–665.
30. Norris JM, Beaty B, Klingensmith G *et al.* Lack of association between early exposure to cow's milk protein and beta-cell autoimmunity. Diabetes Autoimmunity Study in the Young (DAISY). *JAMA* 1996; **276**: 609–614.
31. Vaarala O, Klemetti P, Savilahti E *et al.* Cellular immune response to cow's milk beta-lactoglobulin in patients with newly diagnosed Type 1 diabetes. *Diabetes* 1996; **45**: 178–182.

32. Cavallo MG, Monetini L, Barone F, Pozilli P. Cell mediated immune response to beta casein in recent onset insulin-dependent diabetes: implications for disease pathogenesis. *Lancet* 1996; **348**: 926–928.
33. McEvoy RC, Thomas NM, Ness J. Humoral Immune Markers: Additional Islet Cell Antigens—Important Clues to Pathogenesis or Red Herrings? In Palmer JP (ed.). *Prediction, Prevention and Genetic Counseling in IDDM.* Chichester: Wiley & Sons, 1996; 97–107.
34. Mandrup-Poulsen T, Nerup J. Pathogenesis of childhood diabetes. In Kelnar CJH (ed.). *Childhood and Adolescent Diabetes.* London: Chapman & Hall, 1995; 183–189.
35. Bonifacio E, Cristie MR. Islet cell antigens in the prediction and prevention of insulin-dependent diabetes mellitus. *Ann Med* 1997; **29**: 405–412.
36. Dotta F, Eisenbarth GS. Immunopathogenesis of Type 1 Diabetes in Western Society. In Alberti KGGM, Zimmet P, DeFronzo RA, Keen H (eds). *International Textbook of Diabetes Mellitus*, 2nd edn. Chichester: Wiley, 1997; 97–107.
37. Bonifacio E. Humoral Immune Markers: Islet Cell Antibodies. In Palmer JP (ed.). *Prediction, Prevention and Genetic Counseling in IDDM.* Chichester: Wiley, 1996; 43–61.
38. Greenbaum CJ, Palmer JP. Humoral Immune Markers: Insulin Autoantibodies. In Palmer JP (ed.). *Prediction, Prevention and Genetic Counseling in IDDM.* Chichester: Wiley, 1996; 63–75.
39. Baekkeskov S, Nielsen JH, Marmer B, Bilde T, Ludvigsson J, Lernmark Å. Autoantibodies in newly diagnosed diabetic children immunoprecipitate pancreatic islet cell proteins. *Nature* 1982; **298**: 167–169.
40. Christie MR. Humoral Immune Markers: Antibodies to Glutamic Acid Decarboxylase. In Palmer JP (ed.). *Prediction, Prevention and Genetic Counseling in IDDM.* Chichester: Wiley, 1996; 77–96.
41. Atkinson MA, Bowman MA. T-Cell Markers. In Palmer JP (ed.). *Prediction, Prevention and Genetic Counseling in IDDM.* Chichester: Wiley, 1996; 109–128.
42. Bottazo GF, Dean BM, McNally J, Hackay EH, Swift PGF, Gamble DR. In situ characterization of autoimmune phenomena and expression of HLA molecules in the pancreas in diabetic insulitis. *N Engl J Med* 1985; **313**: 353–360.
43. Foulis AK, Farquharson MA, Harman R. Aberrant expression of class II major histocompatibility complex molecules by B cells and hyperexpression of class I major histocompatibility complex molecules by insulin containing islets in type I (insulin-dependent) diabetes mellitus. *Diabetologia* 1987; **30**: 333–343.
44. Eisenbarth GS. Type 1 diabetes mellitus: a chronic autoimmune disease. *N Engl J Med* 1986; **314**: 1360–1368.

45. Bleich D, Jackson RA, Soeldner JS, Eisenbarth GS. Analysis of metabolic progression to type 1 diabetes in islet cell antibody positive relatives of patients with type 1 diabetes. *Diabetes Care* 1990; **13**: 111–118.
46. Bosi E, Todd I, Pujor-Borell R, Bottazzo GF. Mechanisms of autoimmunity: relevance to the pathogenesis of type 1 (insulin-dependent) diabetes mellitus. *Diabetes Metab Rev* 1987; **3**: 893–924.
47. Muntoni S, Fonte MT, Stoduto S *et al*. Incidence of insulin-dependent diabetes mellitus among Sardinian-heritage children born in Lazio region, Italy. *Lancet* 1997; **349**: 160–162.
48. The Expert Committee on the Diagnosis and Classification of Diabetes Mellitus. Report of the Expert Committee on the Diagnosis and Classification of Diabetes Mellitus. *Diabetes Care* 1997; **20**: 1183–1197.
49. Palmer JP (ed.). *Prediction, Prevention and Genetic Counselling in IDDM*. Chichester: Wiley, 1996.
50. Hahl J, Simell T, Jlonen J, Knip M, Simell O. Costs of predicting IDDM. *Diabetologia* 1998; **41**: 79–85.
51. Eisenbarth GS, Gianani R, Yu L *et al*. Dual-parameters model for prediction of type I diabetes mellitus. *Proc Assoc Am Phys* 1998; **110**: 126–135.
52. Bingley PJ for the ICARUS Group. Interactions of age, islet cell antibodies, insulin autoantibodies and first-phase insulin response in predicting risk of progression to IDDM in ICA relatives: the ICARUS data set. *Diabetes* 1996; **45**: 1720–1728.
53. Tuomilehto J, Wolf E. Primary prevention of diabetes mellitus. *Diabetes Care* 1987; **10**: 238–248.
54. Tuomilehto J, Tuomilehto-Wolf E, Zimmet P, Alberti KGMM, Knowler WC. Primary Prevention of Diabetes Mellitus. In Alberti KGMM, Zimmet P, DeFronzo RA, Keen H (eds). *International Textbook of Diabetes Mellitus*, 2nd edn. Chichester: Wiley, 1997: 1799–1827.
55. Pozzilli P. Present facts and prospects. *Diabet Nutr Metab* 1996; **9**: 306–309.

3

Preventing Type 1 Diabetes in Animal Models

For over 100 years, beginning with Claude Bernard's studies and the pancreatectomy experiments performed by von Mehring and Minkowski, the utilization of animals has brought major contributions to the development of diabetology and its related fields[1–3]. A brilliant example is the discovery of insulin in 1921, which would not have been possible if Paulescu and the Toronto team had not carried out thorough and difficult experimental research[4,5]. Much of our data on the etiology, pathogenesis and treatment of human diabetes would not be available today without the background offered by studies of animal diabetes. The role of experimental work was, and is still, decisive for the progress in the prevention of type 1 diabetes mellitus[6].

3.1   ANIMAL MODELS OF TYPE 1 DIABETES

Usually, these are classified into two groups: induced and sponta-neous models.

3.1.1   Induced Animal Models of Type 1 Diabetes

The principal methods of bringing about experimental type 1 diabetes are listed in Table 3.1.

Table 3.1. The methods of producing type 1 diabetes mellitus in animals

---

Pancreatectomy
Viruses (EMC, meningovirus, Coxsackie virus, etc.)
Chemical agents:
  Alloxan
  Streptozotocin:
    single-dose streptozotocin diabetes
    multiple low-dose streptozotocin diabetes
  Nitrosamines
  Zinc chelating compounds
  Pyriminil
  Others

Adapted from reference 6

Pancreatectomy, already mentioned in dogs, could also be practiced in rats and mice.

The involvement of viruses in the pathogenesis of beta-cell destruction and of type 1 diabetes has been discussed for a long time (see previous chapter). In early studies of the association between viruses and diabetes, viruses were considered as causative factors for diabetes. Today, it is known that some viruses could impede the development of the disease. The viruses most frequently used for the induction of diabetes in mice are encephalomyocarditis virus (EMC) (myocardial strain), meningovirus (clone 2T) and Coxsackie virus (B group)[6,7].

Different chemical factors, especially alloxan and streptozotocin, have been used to produce diabetes in the laboratory. Some details about these substances and about their mechanisms of action were given in Chapter 2.

3.1.2 Spontaneous Animal Models of Type 1 Diabetes

We believe that two main factors are involved in the pathogenesis of type 1 diabetes: genetic susceptibility and the immune system. Only animals which develop spontaneous diabetes can be considered as adequate models for studying the role of these two complementary factors[6]. At present, the most interesting and useful data come from the Bio Breeding (BB) rat and the non-obese diabetic (NOD) mouse as their diabetic syndromes closely resemble human type 1 diabetes[8].

Other animal models with spontaneous type 1 diabetes are the Long–Evans Tokushima Lean (LETL) rat, Chinese hamster, Keeshond dog, Celebes black ape (*Macaca nigra*), some guinea-pig colonies and the New Zealand white rabbit[2,6,8].

3.1.2.1 BB Rat

This animal model was discovered in 1974 by a commercial breeding company (Bio Breeding Laboratories, Ottawa, Ontario, Canada). The diabetic syndrome of the BB rat has many aspects in common with the human disease. The clinical symptoms occur at the age of 3 months, often coinciding with puberty and manifesting as weight loss, polyuria, polydipsia, glycosuria, hyperglycemia and hypoinsulinemia. There is no sex difference regarding the incidence of diabetes. The disorder may progress to ketoacidosis, which often proves to be lethal if exogenous insulin is not administered[9]. The onset of the disease is associated with a pancreatic mononuclear cell infiltrate (insulitis) that is related in degree to the severity of the disease. The process is similar to that of human diabetes with T cells (including both helper and cytotoxic/suppressor subsets), macrophages, NK cells and B lymphocytes present at the onset[8].

Although the precise mode of inheritance of diabetes in BB rats is not well known, the susceptibility for it seems to be associated with the MHC as in human subjects and NOD mice. Cross-breeding experiments have emphasized that the RT1u MHC haplotype is necessary for induction of the disease and this may require the presence of one MHC gene as well as at least two other genes not linked to the MHC[6,8,10]. Diabetes-prone BB rats (BB-DP) maintained in specific pathogen-free (SPF) conditions have a cumulative incidence of diabetes of 60–100%[11].

Both humoral and cellular immunity are involved in the pathogenesis of diabetes in the BB rat. Autoantibodies against islet cell antigens have been described although the BB rat does not have antibodies which produce the ICA reaction on frozen sections. There is an increased frequency of autoantibodies against antigens from other organs such as the thyroid or stomach[11]. It is also interesting to note that GAD antibodies and GAD-reactive T cells have been reported in BB rats as well as in NOD mice[12].

An important characteristic of BB rats is lymphopenia—a complete lack of T lymphocytes at birth—affecting both the $CD4^+$ and $CD8^+$ populations[11]. It has been shown that diabetes could not develop in the absence of lymphopenia although lymphopenia could occur without diabetes[10], although BB rats have been seen to develop diabetes in the absence of lymphopenia or depressed T-cell responses, suggesting that neither abnormality is necessary for the development of diabetes in these animals[13].

3.1.2.2 NOD Mouse

This model was discovered in 1974 in Osaka, Japan. The diabetic syndrome of the NOD mice is similar to that of human subjects, including glycosuria, hyperglycemia and hypoinsulinemia with insulin dependence occurring at about the age of 14 weeks[6]. The insulitis is present in virtually all diabetes-prone NOD mice from about the age of 5 weeks but overt diabetes occurs in only 80% of female and 20% of male mice[14].

In the NOD mouse there are alterations in cellular immunity such as a decreased number of T lymphocytes, decrease in NK cell number and reduced antibody-dependent cell-mediated cytotoxicity. Humoral immunity is also involved. Thus, in prediabetic NOD mice, the existence of ICA, ICSA and IAA has been reported. The disease appears only in those animals in which these antibodies are found. In pancreatic islet infiltrates, helper and cytotoxic T cells can be observed as well as NK cells and other immune cells[8]. It has been shown that at the onset there is a non-destructive peri-insular infiltrate which is characterized by a T-helper type 2 (Th2) associated cytokine pattern and progresses to insular infiltration and beta-cell destruction. This phase is associated with Th1-type immune reactions[15-17]. O'Brien *et al.* have shown that beta-cell apoptosis is responsible for the development of diabetes in the NOD/Lt mouse and that its onset precedes lymphocytic infiltration of the islets[18]. The recently published results of Augstein *et al.*[19] are more consistent with the view that spontaneous beta-cell destruction in the NOD mouse occurs gradually, rather than rapidly just before the onset of diabetes, accounting for the difficulty in securing evidence for short-lived beta-cell apoptosis[19]. Of the immunologic problems under intensive discussion in connection with NOD mice, the putative autoantigens, the effector cells (macrophages, CD4$^+$, CD8$^+$) and the participation of different cytokine subsets (Th1, Th2, IFN-γ, TNF-α) are of special interest[6].

It must be emphasized that research into the genetics of type 1 diabetes in NOD mice is very lively as a result of their importance to the explanation of some of the aspects of the genetics of human diabetes[20]. The genes involved have been provisionally designated *Idd* genes pending their precise categorization. The contribution of the MHC should be emphasized: *Idd1* has been clearly established as the most important component of the susceptibility. This MHC-coded susceptibility involves multiple genes and includes both lack of expression of *Ea* (homologous to DRα in human subjects) and expression of a unique *Ab* locus (histidine as residue number 56 and serine as residue number 57, homologous to "diabetogenic" HLA-DQβ non-aspartic acid 57-containing alleles)[21]. The involvement of some non-MHC genes that are located on many chromosomes has also been brought to light. Different subsets of non-MHC genes are able to interact with a diabetogenic MHC haplotype to bring about the threshold of susceptibility required for the development of diabetes[6,20].

3.2   METHODS OF PREVENTING TYPE 1 DIABETES IN ANIMALS

This subject has been tackled extensively in recent years by many researchers. Interesting and encouraging results have been obtained and some of these have become the basis for projects on preventing type 1 diabetes in humans[22,23].

The existing data will be organized commencing from major stages of the etiopathogenic process (Table 3.2).

3.2.1   Attempts at Genomic Modification

The progress made in transgenic technology has provided a powerful tool for the investigation of the fundamental problems of diabetes[2,6,8,24]. Transgenic mice are created by injecting hybrid genes

Table 3.2. The prevention of type 1 diabetes mellitus in animals (main methods)

Attempts at genomic modification
Influencing environmental factors:
    Infectious agents
    Nutrition
    Stress
Immunotherapeutic procedures:
    Interventions in immune cell subsets
    Islet antigen specific therapy
    Antigen non-specific agents
    Cytokines
    Interventions directed at macrophages
    Thymectomy
    Interventions on the metabolic activity of immune cells
Immunomodulation and tolerance induction:
    Bone marrow transplantation
    Intrathymic islet transplantation
    Cell transfer (including "lymphocyte vaccination")
    Immunomodulating agents
Immunosuppression:
    Irradiation
    Cyclosporine
    Other immunosuppressive drugs
Protection of the beta cells from autoimmune attack:
    Agents affecting beta-cell activity
    Antioxidants
    Inhibitors of nitric oxide synthase

Adapted from reference 6

into the nucleus of fertilized mouse eggs. At present, there is great interest in the production of mouse models to evaluate the selective destruction of the pancreatic beta cells in type 1 diabetes.

It has been shown that the genetic alteration of both MHC class II and class I antigens by transgenic insertion or gene knockout in NOD could protect against diabetes. However, there is some controversy as to how effective these manipulations could be[6,23].

Some studies have demonstrated that plasmid DNA (designated "DNA vaccine") injected into skeletal muscle is picked up by myocytes and subsequently the genes in the plasmid can be expressed for several months and activate the immune system. Using this strategy, Yatokui *et al.* showed that intramuscular injections of DNA expressing GAD 65 (and IL-4) can prevent the development of diabetes by inducing GAD-specific regulatory Th2 cells and can be considered as a new therapeutic approach to type 1 diabetes[25].

3.2.2   Influencing Environmental Factors

The possibility of preventing diabetes with the help of viruses or bacterial products has been reported: for instance, the injection of a lymphocytic choriomeningitis virus prevented insulitis and diabetes in both BB rats and NOD mice[26,27]. This virus infects a subpopulation of lymphocytes and may stimulate the production of suppressor cells or inhibit lymphocytes required for the beta-cell destructive process. Thus, infection of lymphocytes can either protect from or promote the development of diabetes, depending on the strain of virus and the status of the immune system of the host[22]. Infection with other viruses, such as the encephalomyocarditis virus, lactate dehydrogenase virus or mouse hepatitis virus, eliminates the onset of diabetes in NOD mice[22,23]. Complete Freund's adjuvant (containing *Mycobacterium tuberculosis*) and OK 432 (a *Streptococcus pyogenes* A3 preparation) inhibit the development of insulitis and diabetes in BB rats. Similar effects have been seen in NOD mice with the fungal polypeptide LZ-8 and BCG (containing *Mycobacterium bovis*)[22]. More recently, Beales *et al.* have demonstrated that incomplete Freund's adjuvant alone can reduce the incidence of diabetes in the NOD mouse model[28]. An ultraclean environment actually increases the incidence of diabetes.

The connection between nutrition and prevention of animal diabetes has been studied with increasing attention and it has been found that some semi-purified diets containing non-diabetogenic protein sources inhibit the development of diabetes in BB rats[22]. The initial investigations started with casein, but other protein sources such as fish meal, lactalbumin, peanut meal and ground corn are non-diabetogenic also[29]. In contrast, the incidence of diabetes associated with cows' milk whey protein sources is variable in the BB rat[22]. In NOD mice, casein hydrolysate can prevent overt diabetes if it is included early in the diet[30]. However, Paxson *et al.* have noted that neither cows' milk whey proteins in general nor BSA in particular are of significance as etiologic agents in diabetes in NOD mice[31]. Karges *et al.*, in a pilot study for the cows' milk-based IDDM prevention trial, noted that the clinical trial diet effectively protected NOD mice from diabetes, where it affects some T-cell repertoires and allows the development of regulatory cells that interfere with destructive auto-immunity[32]. Fish oil and deficiency of essential fatty acids have shown a protective effect in some studies on diabetes-prone BB rats[22]. 2-Acetyl-4-tetrahydroxybutylimidazole, a widely used food additive, reduced the frequency of diabetes in NOD mice[23,33]. The recent data of Tobia *et al.* indicate that dietary treatment of BB-DP rats with zinc appears to be an effective approach to delaying or preventing the onset of diabetes in genetically predisposed rodents[34]. This finding may suggest further experimental studies regarding dietary means for the preservation of pancreatic function.

Scott *et al.* emphasized that diabetogenic agents in the diet are an essential part of the pathogenesis of diabetes in the BB-DP rats[35]. Diet is also a major factor in determining diabetes outcome in NOD mice and is probably also an important determinant in humans. The influence of food on the expression of diabetes is time- and dose-dependent involving at least two essential elements: (1) changes in the target beta cells, as reflected by altered islet area and antigenicity, followed by (2) a shift in the balance between Th1 and Th2 cells in the tissue undergoing autoimmune attack[35].

Some studies concerning the relationship between stress and the prevention of diabetes have also been carried out[20].

3.2.3 Immunotherapeutic Procedures

This section includes a long list of procedures carried out on the immune system (see Table 3.2). Unfortunately, there is as yet no possibility of separating them in terms of mechanism[6].

A series of interventions directed at immunocyte subsets have been carried out for the purpose of prevention. Initially, antilymphocyte serum was used but later a variety of monoclonal antibodies were found to be just as, or more, effective. In BB rats, antibodies to CD5$^+$, CD8$^+$, NK, CD4$^+$ and to other subsets such as CD2$^+$ have been tried[22,36]. In NOD mice, anti-CD4 antibodies, anti-CD8 antibodies and several other T-cell specific antibodies have been used[22,37]. It is worth noting that monoclonal antibodies to cytokines, receptors and adhesion molecules have also been prepared and used[6].

Ideal immunotherapy for type 1 diabetes would use a precise antigen or even antigenic epitope-specific form of immune unresponsiveness, a therapy which might leave the rest of the immune system intact. There are several antigens that could be candidates for islet antigen-specific treatment in type 1 diabetes: trials with whole islets or islet cells, GAD-65 protein, insulin or heat-shock proteins seem capable of preventing diabetes in NOD mice[23]. Tisch *et al.* have reported that GAD-65 treatment can effectively block disease progression in NOD mice and that protection is mediated through the induction of regulatory CD4$^+$ T cells with a Th2 phenotype[38].

Among "non-specific" agents are complete Freund's adjuvant, BCG vaccine and OK 432[23,39] (these components have already been mentioned in connection with environmental factors). Calcinaro *et al.* suggested a role for IL-4 and IL-10 in complete Freund's adjuvant-induced protection from diabetes in the NOD mouse[40]. A non-specific delay of diabetes onset in the NOD mouse can be produced by IgG2a antibodies[41]. It has also been suggested that exogenous superantigens such as staphylococcal enterotoxin B could prevent the development of autoimmune diabetes in NOD mice[42,43].

The administration of certain cytokines such as TNF-α, IL-1, IL-2 or IL-4 can prevent diabetes in NOD mice[6]. Cailleau *et al.* have shown that IL-1β is a critical effector molecule in NOD mice and that its specific inhibition could be an attractive target for therapeutic intervention[44]. The administration of recombinant IL-4 (rIL-4) prevented diabetes but enhanced pancreatic insulitis[45]. Moritani *et al.* are of the opinion that autoimmune diabetes in NOD mice is not a systemic disease and can be completely prevented by the paracrine TGF-β1 in the islet compartment through protection against CD4$^+$ and CD8$^+$ effector lymphocytes[46]. Brod *et al.* have shown that ingested IFN-α suppressed diabetes in NOD mice and suggest that ingested IFN-α may be an ideal treatment for type 1 diabetes before or immediately after diagnosis[47].

In BB rats, the effects of IL-1, IL-2, TNF-γ and TNF-β have also been tested[6]. Sobel and Newsome have reported that rIFN-γ paradoxically and potently prevents diabetes in BB rats in a dose-dependent fashion by inhibiting islet inflammation. This diabetes-sparing effect occurs even when injections are initiated after the diabetic process has begun[48]. The paradoxical antidiabetogenic effect of gamma-interferon in BB-DP (diabetes-prone) rats was also observed by Nicoletti *et al.*[49]. It has been shown recently that rIFN-α treatment potently prevents diabetes in BB rats by inhibiting the development of insulitis. This effect may have significant implications for the treatment and prevention of type 1 diabetes and for the understanding of the autoimmune process[50].

Some interventions which are specifically addressed at macrophages, cells that play an important role in insulitis, have turned out to be interesting[22,51].

A complete neonatal thymectomy, which causes the systemic elimination of mature thymus-derived T cells, can be successful in preventing diabetes in diabetes-prone rats[52].

Cells of the immune system have a very active metabolism. When they are functionally stimulated, their requirements for energy and biosynthetic substrates increase to sustain their activities. Some experimental data suggest that attenuation of this increase in metabolism (without damaging the integrity of the immune cells) could be another promising preventive measure[22].

3.2.4   Immunomodulation and Induction of Tolerance

Bone marrow and intrathymic islet transplantation have been used as preventive methods in BB-DP rats[6,22].

Transfer of individual and mixed-cell populations have been studied to a large extent both in BB rats and in NOD mice[22,23]. So, for example, it has been demonstrated that a single injection of MHC-compatible spleen cells from Wistar or BB-DR rats can prevent diabetes in BB-DP rats if given early in life[6,53]. Hammond *et al.* have shown that NK T cells prevent diabetes in NOD/Lt mice due to the influence of IL-4 or IL-10[54]. Grafted immunoisolated human benign insulinoma reduces the incidence of diabetes in young NOD mice without abolishing autoimmunity[55].

A therapeutic maneuver, designated "lymphocyte vaccination", in which activated lymphocytes capable of transferring an autoimmune disorder are instead attenuated and administered in vaccine form has been developed[56]. Smerdon *et al.* have shown that a similar procedure applied to NOD mice at 6 weeks of age reduces the incidence of diabetes by 50%[57]. To assess whether this method has potential relevance, in a recent study lymphocyte vaccination was used in NOD mice in 3-weekly doses, commencing in the immediate prediabetic period (age 12 weeks) when insulitis is already advanced and diabetes at onset[58]. Of 30 NOD mice receiving active vaccine (composed of attenuated lymphocytes from diabetic NOD mice) 13 (43.3%) remained non-diabetic to the age of 30 weeks, compared with 2 of 30 (6.7%; $p < 0.01$) mice receiving a control vaccine (composed of attenuated lymphocytes from non-diabetic NOD/B10 mice) and 5 of 26 (19.2%; $p < 0.01$) mice receiving only saline carrier. In an additional group of 10 NOD mice receiving active vaccine weekly between 12 and 30 weeks, 8 remained non-diabetic at the end of the treatment. The delay in the onset of diabetes was accompanied by a reduction in insulitis and, in some cases, a complete absence of infiltrating cells at 30 weeks of age. Immunocytochemistry indicated that, when present, islet infiltrating cells in non-diabetic mice that received active vaccine showed significantly reduced staining for IFN-γ compared with the infiltrate seen in diabetic mice receiving the control vaccine or saline. This study demonstrated that the rapid progression to diabetes typically seen in 12-week-old NOD mice can be delayed by lymphocyte vaccination, supporting the possibility that a vaccine composed of attenuated autologous peripheral blood lymphocytes could be efficient in high-risk first-degree relatives of patients with type 1 diabetes mellitus[58].

The number of substances with immunomodulatory effects which have been tested with the scope of diabetes prevention is increasing[6]. Nicotinamide is a precursor for new nicotinamide adenine dinucleotide synthesis and an inhibitor of poly(ADP-ribose) synthetase and other ADP-ribosyl transferases. It has been proved that nicotinamide has preventive and therapeutic effects on diabetes on NOD mice[23,59]. Various anti-inflammatory agents, an azaspirane compound and dihydroxyvitamin D_3 have also been tested[6,22,23]. Casteels *et al.* have shown that non-hypercalcemic analogs of 1,25-dihydroxyvitamin D_3 administered to NOD mice when the autoimmune disease is already active can prevent clinical diabetes if this therapy is combined with a short induction course of an immunosuppressant such as cyclosporin A[60]. It has also been observed that 1,25-dihydroxyvitamin D_3 restores sensitivity to cyclophosphamide-induced apoptosis in NOD mice and protects against diabetes[61]. Linomide is a potent immunomodulator that has been reported to prevent diabetes and insulitis in NOD mice and to reduce the incidence of some other autoimmune diseases[62]. The phosphodiesterase inhibitors pentoxifylline and rolipram prevent diabetes in NOD mice[63]. Martin *et al.* recently demonstrated that soluble forms of intercellular adhesion molecule-1 inhibit insulitis and onset of autoimmune diabetes[64].

Sulfonylurea compounds have also been evaluated in an effort to develop new and safer methods of prevention. It is known that oral sulfonylureas lower blood glucose levels in type 2 diabetic patients and can induce clinical remissions in new-onset human type 1 diabetes[65]. Attempts at preventing animal diabetes have been carried out with sulfonylurea derivatives of both generations. It has been shown, for example, that tolbutamide reduces the incidence of diabetes mellitus but not of insulitis in NOD mice[66]. On the other hand, glipizide prevents the occurrence of diabetes in BB rats. The mechanism of sulfonylurea-induced prevention could be complex and include metabolic and immunological interventions[67,68].

Glimepiride, a new oral sulfonylurea drug (already on the market as Amaryl) has also been tested for the prevention of diabetes in BB-DP rats[69]. For comparison, at the same time S750181, a sulfonylurea drug with minimal *in vivo* glucose metabolic effects, was evaluated. In addition, the shortest period of sulfonylurea treatment required for prevention was determined. Eighty rats were studied for all treatment periods with 40 receiving a daily oral dosage of glimepiride and 40 receiving a vehicle solution. In study I, with a treatment period of 35–142 days, glimepiride-treated animals showed a 32% incidence of diabetes whereas controls had a diabetes incidence of 55% ($p < 0.04$). In study II, with a treatment period of 60–140 days, glimepiride-treated animals showed a 29% incidence of diabetes vs. 54% in controls ($p < 0.03$) (Figure 3.1.). Further, glimepiride delays diabetes onset ($p < 0.02$). In study III, with a treatment period of 60–100 days, glimepiride-treated rats presented a 17% overall diabetes incidence at 170 days of age vs. 43% in controls ($p < 0.01$). In study IV, with a treatment period of 60–140 days, S750181-treated animals showed a 38% diabetes incidence and the control group had a 43% incidence. There was no significant delaying or preventive effect in the S750181 group. The severity of islet inflammation was examined to determine the influence of glimepiride on the autoimmune events. In study I,

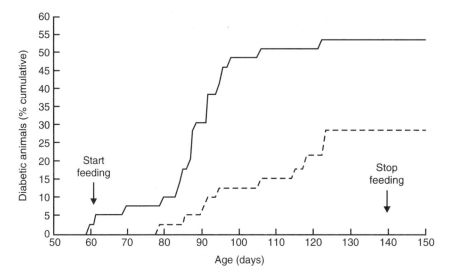

Figure 3.1. Effect of oral glimepiride 200 mg/kg/day (- - - -) on incidence of diabetes in BB rats (study II). (———) Control. Adapted from reference 69

islet histology from treated and non-diabetic animals demonstrated that glimepiride-treated rats had a lower severity of insulitis than that of the control rats ($p < 0.023$). The studies mentioned above showed that: (a) glimepiride has diabetes preventive action; (b) a shorter treatment period of only 40 days can be efficient; and (c) glimepiride decreases the severity of islet inflammation. It has thus been confirmed that sulfonylureas are effective in preventing diabetes in BB rats and that their mechanism of action appears to be related to dampening of autoimmune responses[69,70].

3.2.5 Immunosuppression

Total lymphoid irradiation was one of the earlier interventions that led to the prevention of diabetes in BB rats[71].

Cyclosporine administration has been tried in both BB rats and NOD mice[22,23]. The best results in rats were obtained with continuous administration of cyclosporine using dosage schedules that resulted in trough plasma levels between 100 and 300 ng/ml. The protective effect of cyclosporine against diabetes in animals was a prototype for the testing of this compound in humans[6].

The list of other immunosuppressive agents which have been used in animal diabetes prevention includes azathioprine, cyclophosphamide, FK-506, ciamexone, fusidic acid, rapamycin, cortisone acetate, mycophenolate mofetil, deoxypergualin and a new class of immuno-conjugates[22,23]. Of the recently tested agents are the immunosuppressive agent FTY 720 and the so-called "disintegrins" isolated from the venom of various vipers[72,73].

3.2.6 Protection of the Beta Cells from Autoimmune Attack

As far back as 1985, it was discovered that exogenous insulin given at a young age markedly reduced the incidence of diabetes in BB-DP rats[74]. It has been suggested that the protective effect of insulin may be a result of an altered functional, quiescent, state of the beta cells, termed "beta-cell rest". Numerous studies since then have given a large amount of consideration to this idea and have enabled its application in humans[6]. The investigators also verified that prophylactic insulin therapy might prevent diabetes in NOD mice. The mice were injected with protamine zinc pork insulin from weaning until 6 months; the treatment significantly reduced the frequency of diabetes and pancreatic insulitis[23,75]. In a more unusual but practical approach, the oral administration of porcine insulin was tested in NOD mice. Insulin was given orally twice a week for 5 weeks and then weekly until 1 year of age. Despite having no demonstrable metabolic action, the treatment reduced the severity of islet infiltration and the incidence of diabetes[76]. I have mentioned the attempts with oral insulin in order to continue the discussion about the preventive role of insulin, but the mechanisms of action in the case of oral insulin differ.

Vlahos *et al.* have shown that diazoxide is as potent as insulin in preventing the appearance of diabetes in BB rats while glyburide has no effect[77]. Buschard *et al.* reported that neonatal stimulation of beta cells in BB-DP rats with glucagon or arginine reduced the subsequent onset of diabetes from 65 to 20–23%[78].

A significant number of antioxidant agents have been used to prevent diabetes in NOD mice and BB rats. Some examples are probucol, α-tocopherol, Max EPA, a mixture of free-radical scavengers, lazaroid and lipoic acid[22,23,79].

There has been a virtual explosion of interest in the role of nitric oxide as a mediator of beta-cell damage[22]. Inhibitors of nitric oxide synthase also have diabetes preventive effects. Among these are the arginine analogs and aminguanidine[80,81].

3.3 CONCLUSIONS

The variety of the ways of preventing type 1 diabetes mellitus in animal models is impressive. For this reason, clear documentation is very hard to achieve. Practicing physicians are more and more attentive to the signals emanating from experimental diabetes. Those who have truly fought for the development of preventive strategies destined for use in human type 1 diabetes have a large data base and very attractive sources of inspiration.

REFERENCES

1. Krall LP, Levine RL, Barnett DM. The History of Diabetes. In Kahn CR, Weir GC (eds). *Joslin's Diabetes Mellitus*, 13th edn. Philadelphia: Lea & Febiger, 1994; 1–14.
2. Karasik A, Hattori M. Use of Animal Models in the Study of Diabetes. In Kahn CR, Weir GC (eds). *Joslin's Diabetes Mellitus*, 13th edn. Philadelphia: Lea & Febiger, 1994; 317–350.
3. Shafrir E. Editor's preface: Introduction to Lessons from Animal Diabetes VI. In Shafrir E (ed). *Lessons from Animal Diabetes VI. 75th Anniversary of the Insulin Discovery*. Boston: Birkhausen, 1996; IX–X.
4. Paulesco NC. Action de l'extrait pancréatique injecté dans le sang, chez un animal diabétique. *CR Soc Biol* 1921; **85**: 555–559.
5. Banting FG, Best CH. The internal secretion of the pancreas. *Lab Clin Med* 1922; **7**: 251–266.
6. Cheţa D. Animal models of type I (insulin-dependent) diabetes mellitus. *J Pediatr Endocrinol Metab* 1998; **11**: 11–19.
7. Szopa TM, Titchener PA, Portwood ND, Taylor KW. Diabetes mellitus due to viruses—some recent developments. *Diabetologia* 1993; **36**: 687–695.

8. Bone AJ, Gwillian DJ. Animal Models of Insulin-Dependent Diabetes Mellitus. In Pickup JC, Williams G (eds). *Textbook of Diabetes*, 2nd edn. Oxford: Blackwell Science, 1997; 16.1–16.6.
9. Nakhooda AF, Like AA, Chappel CI, Murray FT, Marliss EB. The spontaneously diabetic Wistar rat. Metabolic and morphologic studies. *Diabetes* 1976; **26**: 100–112.
10. Guttmann RD, Colle E, Michel F, Seemayer T. Spontaneous diabetes syndrome in the rat. II. T lymphopenia and its association with clinical disease and pancreatic infiltration. *J Immunol* 1983; **109**: 2264–2266.
11. Pettersson A, Jacob H, Lernmark Å. Lessons from the Animal Models: The BB Rat. In Palmer JP (ed.). *Prediction, Prevention and Genetic Counseling in IDDM*. Chichester: Wiley, 1996; 181–200.
12. Faulkner-Jones BE, French MB, Schmidli RS *et al.* Expression of glutamic acid decarboxylase (GAD) and its role as an autoantigen in insulin-dependent diabetes. In Shafrir E (ed.). *Lessons from Animal Diabetes VI. 75th Anniversary the Insulin Discovery.* Boston: Birkhausen, 1996; 1–32.
13. Varey AM, Dean BM, Walker R, Bone AJ, Baird JD, Cooke A. Immunological responses of the BB rat colony in Edinburgh. *Immunology* 1987; **60**: 131–134.
14. Makino S, Kunimoto K, Muraoka Y, Mizushima Y, Katagiri K, Tochino Y. Breeding of a non-obese, diabetic strain of mice. *Exp Anim* 1980; **29**: 1–13.
15. Rothe H, Faust A, Shade U *et al.* Cyclophosphamide treatment of female non-obese mice causes enhanced expression of inducible nitric oxide synthase and interferon-gamma, but not of interleukin-4. *Diabetologia* 1994; **37**: 1154–1158.
16. Rabinovitch A. Immunoregulatory and cytokine imbalances in the pathogenesis of IDDM–therapeutic intervention by immunostimulation? *Diabetes* 1994; **43**: 613–621.
17. Hartman B, Bellmann K, Ghiea I, Kleemann R, Kolb H. Oral insulin for diabetes prevention in NOD mice: potentiation by enhancing Th_2 cytokine expression in the gut through bacterial adjuvant. *Diabetologia* 1997; **40**: 902–909.
18. O'Brien BA, Harmon BV, Cameron DP, Allan DJ. Apoptosis is the mode of β-cell death responsible for the development of IDDM in the nonobese diabetic (NOD) mouse. *Diabetes* 1997; **46**: 750–757.
19. Augstein P, Elefanty AG, Allison J, Harrison LC. Apoptosis and beta-cell destruction in pancreatic islets of NOD mice with spontaneous and cyclophosphamide-accelerated diabetes. *Diabetologia* 1998; **41**: 1381–1388.
20. Leiter EH. Lessons from the Animal Models: The NOD Mouse. In Palmer JP (ed.). *Prediction, Prevention and Genetic Counseling in IDDM*. Chichester: Wiley, 1996; 201–226.

21. Todd JA, Acha-Orbea H, Bell JI *et al.* A molecular basis for MHC class II-associated autoimmunity. *Science* 1988; **240**: 1003–1009.
22. Yale J-F, Scott FW, Marliss EB. Lessons from the Animal Models: BB Rat. In Palmer JP (ed.). *Prediction, Prevention and Genetic Counseling in IDDM.* Chichester: Wiley, 1996; 317–347.
23. Shimada A, Charlton B, Fathman CG. Lessons from Animal Models: NOD Mouse. In Palmer JP (ed.). *Prediction, Prevention and Genetic Counseling in IDDM.* Chichester: Wiley, 1996: 349–368.
24. Shafrir E. Animals with Diabetes: Progress in the Understanding of Diabetes Through Study of its Pathogenesis in Animal Models. In Alberti KGMM, Krall LP (eds). *The Diabetes Annual/6.* Amsterdam: Elsevier, 1991; 634–663.
25. Yatokui M, Shimada A, Takei I, Kasuga A *et al.* Suppressive effect on diabetes development in autoimmune diabetic mice by intramuscular injection of plasmid DNA expressing GAD and IL-4. *Diabetes* 1998; **47** (Suppl 1): A224.
26. Dryberg T, Schwimmbeck PL, Oldstone MBA. Inhibition of diabetes in BB rats by virus infection. *J Clin Invest* 1988: **81**: 928–931.
27. Oldstone MB. Prevention of type I diabetes in nonobese diabetic mice by virus infection. *Science* 1988; **239**: 500–502.
28. Beales PE, Liddi R, Matta G, Webb GP, Pozilli P. Incomplete Freund's adjuvant protects NOD mice from Type 1 diabetes. *Diabetologia* 1998; **41** (Suppl 1): A90.
29. Scott FW. Food, Diabetes and Immunology. In Forse RA, Bell SJ, Blackburn GL, Kabbash LG (eds). *Diet, Nutrition and Immunity.* Boca Raton: CRC Press, 1994; 71–92.
30. Elliot RB, Reddy SN, Bibby NJ, Kida K. Dietary prevention of diabetes in the non-obese diabetic mouse. *Diabetologia* 1983; **31**: 62–64.
31. Paxson JA, Weber JG, Kulczycki A Jr. Cow's milk-free diet does not prevent diabetes in NOD mice. *Diabetes* 1997; **46**: 1711–1717.
32. Karges W, Hammond-Mckibben D, Cheung RK *et al.* Immunological aspects of nutritional diabetes prevention in NOD mice: a pilot study for the cow's milk-based IDDM prevention trial. *Diabetes* 1997; **46**: 557–564.
33. Mandel TE, Koulmanda M, Mackay IR. Prevention of spontaneous and cyclophosphamide-induced diabetes in non-obese diabetic (NOD) mice with oral 2-acetyl-4-tetrahydroxybutylimidazole (THI), a component of caramel coloring III. *Clin Exp Immunol* 1992; **88**: 414–419.
34. Tobia MH, Zdanowicz MM, Wingertzahn MA, McHeffey-Atkinson B, Slonim AE, Wapnir RA. The role of dietary zinc in modifying the onset and severity of spontaneous diabetes in the BB Wistar rat. *Molec Genet Metab* 1998; **63**: 205–213.

35. Scott FW, Cloutier HE, Kleeman R *et al.* Potential mechanisms by which ceratin foods promote or inhibit the development of spontaneous diabetes in BB rats: dosage, timing, early effect on islet area and switch in infiltrate from Th1 to Th2 cells. *Diabetes* 1997; **46**: 589–598.
36. Like AA, Biron CA, Weringer EJ, Byman K, Sroczynski , Guberski L. Prevention of diabetes in Bio Breeding/Worcester rats with monoclonal antibodies that recognize T lymphocytes or natural killer cells. *J Exp Med* 1986; **164**: 1145–1159.
37. Hayward AR, Shriber M, Cooke A, Woldmann H. Prevention of diabetes but not insulitis in NOD mice injected with antibody to CD4. *J Autoimmun* 1993; **6**: 301–310.
38. Tisch R, Liblau Y, Yang X-D, Liblau P, McDevitt HO. Induction of GAD65-specific regulatory T-cells inhibits ongoing autoimmune diabetes in nonobese diabetic mice. *Diabetes* 1998; **47**: 894–899.
39. Shehadeh N, Calcinaro F, Bradley BJ, Bruchlim I, Vardi P, Lafferty KJ. Effect of adjuvant therapy on development of diabetes in mouse and man. *Lancet* 1994; **343**: 706–707.
40. Calcinaro F, Gambelunghe G, Lafferty KJ. Protection from autoimmune diabetes by adjuvant therapy in the non-obese diabetic mouse: the role of interleukin-4 and interleukin-10. *Immunol Cell Biol* 1997; **75**: 467–471.
41. Todd I, Davenport C, Topping JH, Wood PJ. IgG2a antibodies non-specifically delay the onset of diabetes in NOD mice. *Autoimmunity* 1998; **27**: 209–211.
42. Lee M, Jun HS, Lim HVM, Yoon JW. Molecular mechanisms for the prevention of autoimmune IDDM by treatment with a superantigen in NOD mice. *Diabetologia* 1997; **40** (Suppl 1): A66.
43. Schiffenbauer J, Xie T, Clare-Salzler M, Atkinson MA. The effect of superantigen administration on the natural history of IDD in NOD mice. *Diabetologia* 1997; **40** (Suppl 1): A67.
44. Cailleau C, Diu-Hercend A, Ruuth E, Westwood R, Carnaud C. Treatment with neutralizing antibodies specific for IL-1β prevents cyclophosphamide-induced diabetes in nonobese diabetic mice. *Diabetes* 1997; **46**: 937–940.
45. Tominaga Y, Nagata M, Yasuda H *et al.* Administration of IL-4 prevents autoimmune diabetes but enhances pancreatic insulitis in NOD mice. *Clin Immunol Immunopathol* 1998; **86**: 209–218.
46. Moritani M, Yoshimoto K, Wong SF *et al.* Abrogation of autoimmune diabetes in nonobese diabetic mice and protection against effector lymphocytes by transgenic paracrine TGF-beta 1. *J Clin Invest* 1998; **102**: 499–506.
47. Brod SA, Malone M, Darcan S, Papolla M, Nelson L. Ingested interferon α suppresses Type I diabetes in non-obese diabetic mice. *Diabetologia* 1998; **41**: 1227–1232.

48. Sobel DO, Newsome J. Gamma interferon prevents diabetes in the BB rat. *Clin Diag Lab Immunol* 1997; **4**: 764–768.
49. Nicoletti F, Zaccone P, DiMarco R *et al.* Paradoxical antidiabetogenic effect of gamma-interferon in DP-BB rats. *Diabetes* 1998; **47**: 32–38.
50. Sobel DO, Creswell K, Yoon JW, Holterman D. Alpha interferon administration paradoxically inhibits the development of diabetes in BB rats. *Life Sci* 1998; **62**: 1293–1302.
51. Oschilewski U, Kiesel U, Kolb H. Administration of silica prevents diabetes in BB rats. *Diabetes* 1985; **34**: 197–199.
52. Like AA, Kislauskis E, Williams RM, Rossini AA. Neonatal thymectomy prevents spontaneous diabetes mellitus in the BB/W rat. *Science* 1982: **216**: 644–646.
53. Burstein D, Mordes JP, Greiner DL *et al.* Prevention of diabetes in BB/Wor rat by single transfusion of spleen cells parameters that affect degree of protection. *Diabetes* 1989; **38**: 24–30.
54. Hammond KJL, Poulton LD, Palmisano LJ, Silveira PA, Godfrey DI, Baxter AG. Alpha/beta-T cell receptors (TCR) +CD4⁻ CD8⁻ (NKT) thymocytes prevent insulin-dependent diabetes mellitus in nonobese diabetic (NOD)/Lt mice by the influence of interleukin (IL)-4 and/or IL-10. *J Exp Med* 1998; **187**: 1047–1056.
55. Fakir M, Penformis A, Elian N, Cugnenc PH, Altman JJ. Grafted immuno-isolated human benign insulinoma reduces the incidence of diabetes in young NOD mice without abolishing the auto-immunity. *Int J Artific Organs* 1997; **20**: 637–643.
56. Ben-Nun A, Wekerle H, Cohen IR. Vaccination against autoimmune encephalomyelitis with T lymphocyte line cells reactive against myelic basic protein. *Nature* 1981; **292**: 60–61.
57. Smerdon RA, Peakman H, Hussain MJ, Vergani D. Lymphocyte vaccination prevents spontaneous diabetes in the non-obese diabetic mouse. *Immunology* 1993; **80**: 498–501.
58. Gearon CL, Hussain MJ, Vergani D, Peakman M. Lymphocyte vaccination protects prediabetic non-obese diabetic mice from developing diabetes mellitus. *Diabetologia* 1997; **40**: 1388–1395.
59. Yamada K, Nonaka K, Hanafusa T, Miyazaki A, Toyashima H, Tarui S. Preventive and therapeutic effects of large-dose nicotinamide injections on diabetes associated with insulitis. An observation in nonobese diabetic (NOD) mice. *Diabetes* 1982; **31**: 749–753.
60. Casteels KM, Mathieu C, Waer M *et al.* Prevention of type I diabetes in nonobese diabetic mice by late intervention with nonhypercalcemic analogs of 1,25-dihydroxyvitamin D3 in combination with a short induction course of cyclosporin A. *Endocrinology* 1998; **139**: 95–102.
61. Casteels K, Waer M, Bouillon R *et al.* 1,25-Dihydroxyvitamin D3 restores sensitivity to cyclophosphamide-induced apoptosis in non-obese diabetic

(NOD) mice and protects against diabetes. *Clin Exp Immunol* 1998; **112**: 181–187.

62. Hartoft-Nielsen M-L, Kaas A, Rasmussen ÅK, Feldt-Rasmussen U, Buschard K. Linomide does not prevent autoimmune thyroiditis in NOD mice. *Diabetologia* 1998; **41** (Suppl 1): A103.

63. Liang L, Beshay E, Prud'homme GJ. The phosphodiesterase inhibitors pentoxyfilline and rolipram prevent diabetes in NOD mice. *Diabetes* 1998; **47**: 570–575.

64. Martin S, Heidenthal E, Schulte B, Rothe H, Kolb H. Soluble forms of intercellular adhesion molecule-1 inhibit insulitis and onset of autoimmune diabetes. *Diabetologia* 1998; **41**: 1298–1303.

65. Charles MA, Selam JL, Chan E, Woertz L, Robinson M, Lozano J. The effects of intensive insulin treatment and glipizide upon remission induction and endogenous insulin secretion in new onset type 1 diabetes: a randomized trial. *Diabetes* 1991; **40** (Suppl 1): 57A.

66. Williams AJK, Beales PE, Krug J *et al.* Tolbutamide reduces the incidence of diabetes mellitus, but not insulitis in the non-obese-diabetic mouse. *Diabetologia* 1993; **36**: 487–492.

67. Chan E, Hosszufalusi N, Charles MA. The use of glipizide to prevent diabetes in the BB rat. *Diabetes* 1991; **40** (Suppl 1): 116A.

68. Takei S, Cheţa D, Hosszufalusi N, Chan E, Charles MA. The mechanism of sulphonylurea-induced diabetes prevention in the BB rat. *Clin Res* 1992; **40**: 106A.

69. Cheţa DM, Lim J, Chan EK, Kunakorn T, Charles MA. Glimepiride-induced prevention of diabetes and autoimmune events in the BB rat: revised. *Life Sci* 1995; **57**: 2281–2290.

70. Pan J, Chan EK, Cheţa D, Schranz V, Charles MA. The effects of nicotinamide and glimepiride on diabetes prevention in BB rats. *Life Sci* 1995; **57**: 1525–1532.

71. Rossini AA, Slavin S, Woda BA, Geisberg M, Like AA, Mordes JP. Total lymphoid irradiation prevents diabetes mellitus in the Bio-Breeding/Worcester (BB/W) rat. *Diabetes* 1984; **36**: 543–547.

72. Suzuki K, Yan H, Li XK, Amemiya H, Suzuki S, Hiromitsu K. Prevention of experimentally induced autoimmune type I diabetes in rats by the new immunosuppressive reagent FTY 720. *Transplant Proc* 1998; **30**: 1044–1045.

73. Brando C, Marcinkiewicz C, Goldman B, Che Q, Niewiarowski S. Effect of disintegrins on lymphocyte infiltration of Langerhans islets in NOD mice. *Diabetes* 1998; **47** (Suppl 1): A224.

74. Gotfredsen CF, Buschard K, Frandsen EK. Reduction of diabetes incidence of BB-Wistar rats by early prophylactic insulin treatment of diabetes-prone animals. *Diabetologia* 1985; **28**: 933–935.

75. Atkinson MA, Maclaren NK, Luchetta R. Insulitis and diabetes in NOD mice reduced by prophylactic insulin therapy. *Diabetes* 1990; **39**: 933–937.

76. Zhang ZJ, Davidson L, Eisenbarth G, Weiner HL. Suppression of diabetes in nonobese diabetic mice by oral administration of porcine insulin. *Proc Natl Acad Sci USA* 1991; **88**: 10252–10256.

77. Vlahos WD, Seemayer TA, Yale J-F. Diabetes prevention in BB rats by inhibition of endogenous insulin secretion. *Metabolism* 1991; **40**: 825–829.

78. Buschard K, Jorgensen M, Aaen K, Bock T, Josefsen N. Prevention of diabetes mellitus in BB rats by neonatal stimulation of B cells. *Lancet* 1990; **335**: 134–135.

79. Fleschner I, Maruta K, Burkart V, Kawai K, Kolb H, Kiesel V. Effects of radical scavengers on the development of experimental diabetes. *Diabetes Res Clin Pract* 1992; **18**: 11–16.

80. Wu G. Nitric oxide synthesis and the effect of aminoguanidine and N^G-monomethil-L-arginine on the onset of diabetes in the spontaneously diabetic BB rat. *Diabetes* 1995; **44**: 360–364.

81. Holstad M, Jansson L, Sandler S. Inhibition of nitric oxide formation by aminoguanidine: an attempt to prevent insulin-dependent diabetes mellitus. *Gen Pharmacol* 1997; **29**: 697–700.

4

Prevention Projects for Human Type 1 Diabetes

4.1 GENERAL ASPECTS

The primary prevention of type 1 diabetes could be realized by either a high-risk or a population-based approach. The high-risk approach involves identification of susceptible individuals (e.g. first- and second-degree relatives of the patients) and then prevention of onset of the disease by influencing the genetic susceptibility or the precipitating environmental factors. The population-based approach is more difficult and could be aimed at modification of lifestyle or the elimination of those environmental determinants that are known to be risk factors for type 1 diabetes[1,2].

Although the susceptibility to type 1 diabetes is inherited, the principal problem in its prevention using the high-risk approach is that only 12–15% of the disease occurs in families. The major proportion of type 1 diabetes—about 85%—occurs in a sporadic fashion. As was shown in Chapter 2, the genetic predisposition to type 1 diabetes is conferred mainly by genes in the HLA region, which is located on the short arm of chromosome 6. In addition, there is contribution from some non-HLA genetic factors (their exact role remains to be established in the future). There is as yet no possibility for gene manipulation or gene therapy in human subjects with regard to type 1 diabetes[2].

Here are some observations related to environmental factors. Although a significant number of common viruses (such as mumps, Coxsackie B group and rubella) have been implicated in the development of type 1 diabetes, this disease is not a clear result of viral infection. However, the cost and benefits of a theoretical vaccine for diabetes have been estimated[3]. It was calculated that vaccination of the entire population would be more efficient than that of only high-risk subjects: the incidence of type 1 diabetes could be reduced annually by 29% and the annual costs by 18%[2].

There is a rapid growth in the volume of information regarding the connections between breastfeeding and cows' milk proteins and type 1 diabetes[4,5]. Based on this, dietary intervention trials have been planned for infants with a high genetic risk of type 1 diabetes in order to explore the effect of the avoidance of dietary cows' milk in preventing the disease[6-9]. Until some firm conclusions have been made, it is prudent to recommend a long duration of breastfeeding, not only for possible prevention of type 1 diabetes but also for many other reasons[2]. If we take into consideration some economic, social and cultural characteristics of the contemporary world (the growth in the level of urbanization, the greater involvement of young women in professional life, the increase in the levels of stress, the preoccupation with personal aesthetics etc.), it is evident that insistence on normal breastfeeding is one of the simpler methods of reducing the risk for type 1 diabetes (and other disorders).

Nitrosamines are toxic substances found in the rodenticide vacor and in streptozotocin. There is convincing evidence for the diabetogenic role of frequent intake of nitrosamine-rich food and of an increased content of nitrates in drinking water[10,11], avoidance of which may also be considered an important preventive measure[2]. Nevertheless, exposed subjects should be properly informed of the risk.

The specific aim of primary prevention of type 1 diabetes mellitus is to find ways to hamper the beta-cell destruction process or to promote the generation of new islet cells from pancreatic duct cells, perhaps through specific interventions on the immune system[12-16]. The field is changing quickly and it is expected that intervention methods for the prevention of type 1 diabetes will increase[17].

In 1990, the US National Institutes of Health organized a workshop to discuss the prevention of type 1 diabetes. The position statement, which was improved in 1994, contains the following points[18].

1. Sufficient data exists to warrant studies for the prevention of type 1 diabetes.
2. Intervention to prevent type 1 diabetes should be attempted only in the context of defined clinical studies under supervision of the Institutional Review Board.
3. Intervention studies for the prevention of type 1 diabetes are best accomplished by randomized control studies.
4. A registry of intervention studies should be maintained and all planned studies should be reported by a coordinating body.

In addition, it was mentioned in the statement that screening of any population outside the context of defined research studies should be discouraged[2]. It was also emphasized that prevention trials should be accompanied from the beginning by a conscientious psychological supervision of probands in order to better understand the impact of this new field of medical intervention on the individual as well as to provide a support network for those unable to cope with this challenge[8].

A number of methods for the prevention of human type 1 diabetes which have aroused (or are arousing) special interest from the scientific and practical point of view are reviewed in the rest of this chapter.

4.2 NICOTINAMIDE

The use of certain substances for the purposes of prevention must be scrutinized for biological plausibility, safety and acceptability. Nicotinamide is an attractive agent as it has been in use clinically for a long time without apparent harmful effects[19].

4.2.1 Pharmacology

Nicotinamide is part of the family of B vitamins. Its deficiency leads to pellagra, which is characterized by abnormalities in the skin, gastrointestinal tract and nervous system. The recommended daily intake is 0.30 mg/kg/day.

Nicotinamide is derived from nicotinic acid by amidation of the carboxyl group. It carries out some of the most important functions in the body after being converted into NAD^+ in the liver. It is metabolized into N-methyl nicotinamide which passes further into N-methyl-2-pyridone-5-carboxamide and N-methyl-4-pyridone-3-carboxamide. These three metabolites are excreted in the urine and urinary N-methyl nicotinamide can be determined as a measure of drug compliance[20].

Nicotinamide is available in solution for injection and regular or slow-release formulated tablets. It is absorbed in all sections of the intestine and is distributed in all tissues. There is evidence that nicotinamide accumulates in the pancreatic islets; islet concentrations may be 100–1000 times higher than in the blood.

Adverse effects in humans at doses of 3–12 g/day have been reported: rashes, hives, dry hair, soreness of the mouth, nausea and vomiting, fatigue and headache amongst others.

Attention has been drawn to the fact that short-term administration of nicotinamide causes insulin resistance and a fall in the constant for glucose disappearance in ICA-positive relatives[21]. For this reason, it was recommended that at least one subgroup of subjects enrolled in clinical trials to prevent type 1 diabetes undergo regular measurements of both insulin sensitivity and insulin secretion[22]. This subgroup should be randomly assigned and large enough for statistical analysis to interpret properly the changes in insulin secretion that may be seen in the intervention trials as a whole[21].

4.2.2   Action of Nicotinamide on Destruction of Beta Cells

The importance of free radicals as effectors of the autoimmune attack on pancreatic beta cells has already been emphasized. Free oxygen radicals and nitric oxide radicals cause DNA strand breaks. The repair process involves the activation of the nuclear enzyme poly(ADP–ribose) polymerase (P[ADPR]P). In this process, the enzyme binds covalently to nucleic proteins to produce poly(ADP-ribose), using nicotinamide adenine dinucleotide (NAD) as a substrate. By inhibiting P(ADPR)P and the enzyme NADase (which breaks down NAD), and by repleting NAD stores, nicotinamide may prevent cellular NAD depletion and death.

Nicotinamide also inhibits cytokine-induced islet nitric oxide production and has other biochemical actions that are compatible with modern concepts of the molecular mechanism leading to beta-cell destruction[19,21,22].

4.2.3 Animal Studies

Large doses of nicotinamide administered immediately before, or within 1 hour of, the intravenous or intraperitoneal injection of streptozotocin have prevented beta-cell damage and diabetes[19,23]. It has also been demonstrated that pre- and postnatal treatment with nicotinamide prevents the development of insulin deficiency in strep-tozotocin-treated newborn rats[24].

Nicotinamide given daily as a subcutaneous injection from the age of 80 days prevented diabetes in NOD mice[25]. The same effect could be obtained using a 1% solution of the vitamin in lieu of drinking water from weaning or 60 days of age. Nicotinamide is ineffective if given too late or in lower doses.

Studies of nicotinamide in BB rats have given contradictory results. After analyzing a number of studies, Pan *et al.* arrived at the conclusion that the timing of nicotinamide administration is very important. The successful preventive studies were carried out on older animals (> 40 days of age) and with short-term interventions (< 80 days). The tolerance of nicotinamide treatment was poor when used in young animals, as shown by a lower body weight and difficulty in feeding. When nicotinamide was used in older rats for a shorter time, no loss of body weight was observed[22].

4.2.4 Human Studies

The preliminary results of a general population study have already been reported[26,27]. This study involved a population of about 81 000 children aged 5–7 at time of admission to the trial (the entire population of that age group of the city available at the time the trial was carried out). Some 33 000 of these children were randomly selected to be tested for islet cell antibodies; of these 20 000 agreed to be part of the test and 13 000 did not. The other 48 000 constituted the control group. Those with persistent islet cell antibodies of 20 or more

JDF units as well as those with 10 units and impaired first-phase insulin release were offered treatment with nicotinamide.

In the control group (48 335 subjects), after a mean follow-up time of 5.2 years, 55 cases of type 1 diabetes were seen—which meant a diabetes incidence of 21/100 000 per year. In the group refusing to be tested (13 463 subjects), 10 cases of diabetes were seen after a mean follow-up time of 4.2 years—a diabetes incidence of 17.7/100 000 per year. In the tested group (20 195 subjects), six cases of diabetes were seen, representing a diabetes incidence of 7.1/100 000 per year after a mean follow-up time of 4.2 years. The maximum follow-up time was only 6 years, so it is far from certain that the results obtained would have remained constant in the long term[19].

Other studies, albeit of smaller size, have produced some interesting data. In one such study, 22 children less than 16 years of age were drawn from two centers on the basis of having high levels of ICA (80 or more) units and a degree of impairment of first-phase insulin response. Of these, eight were untreated and developed diabetes within 5 years. The others were treated daily with 150–300 mg nicotinamide for every year of age. After a similar period of follow up, about half had developed the disease. The subjects were not randomized and the treatment was not blind[28]. In an extension of this study, a larger cohort of subjects who were relatives of all ages with ICA levels of 20 or more JDF units received nicotinamide and their diabetes outcome was compared with that of two large untreated cohorts. A high degree of protection seemed apparent[19,26].

In another study, three subjects, all with high ICA and IAA levels as well as insulin release below the third percentile, did not apparently benefit from nicotinamide compared with other subjects having the same characteristics[29].

The IMDIAB group from Italy arrived at the conclusion that nicotinamide is equally effective at doses of 25 or 50 mg/kg body weight in maintaining residual beta-cell secretion 6 months after diagnosis in patients with type 1 diabetes[30]. The same group has shown that BCG vaccine has no additional therapeutic value compared with nicotinamide[31].

Large double-blind placebo-controlled investigations on the preventive efficiency of nicotinamide in first-degree relatives with ICA $\geq$ 20 units have been organized in Europe and North America[19]. The European Nicotinamide Diabetes Intervention Trial (ENDIT) set out to screen 40 000 first-degree relatives of subjects who developed type 1 diabetes before the age of 20 years with the aim of recruiting 528 high-risk relatives to a 5-year randomized placebo-controlled trial of nicotinamide[32]. Recruits were aged 5–40 years, non-diabetic by oral glucose tolerance test (OGTT) positive for ICA on two occasions with one value ≥ 20 JDF units. The end-point was the development of diabetes. By December 1996, 449 individuals had been randomized in 16 countries. Of these, 62% were below 20 years of age, 48% were females, 29% were parents, 59% siblings and 10% children. ICAs were ≥ 80 JDF units in 29% of cases, 55% had antibodies to GAD, 38% antibodies to IA-2 and 29% antibodies to insulin ≥ 99th percentile of 3000 schoolchildren. A proportion of 43% had at least two antibodies ≥ 99th percentile in addition to ICA. OGTT was normal in 88% and impaired glucose tolerance was present in 12%. Of 263 intravenous glucose tolerance tests (IVGTT) analyzed, 17% had first-phase insulin release $(1' + 3'$ insulin) < 50 mU/1. Subjects under 20 years of age had more risk markers than those of 20 years or older. Of those recruited, 30 developed diabetes and 35 withdrew from the trial. Almost all drop-outs occurred within the first 6 months of the study and the main reasons were difficulty with swallowing tablets (children) or non-compliance. Recruitment ended in 1997 with study completion in 2002. The authors felt that multinational interventional collaborative studies were feasible in preclinical type 1 diabetes. Simple robust entry criteria are essential. ICAs have proved their value, but enrolment in future trials will probably be based on multiple antibody testing[32,33].

4.3   CYCLOSPORINE, AZATHIOPRINE AND CORTICOSTEROIDS

The first works concerning the immunotherapy of human type 1 diabetes appeared in the early 1980s[34,35]. It could be said that immunosuppression with cyclosporine and azathioprine for patients with newly diagnosed diabetes remain the most rigorously tested approaches thus far. At present, however, the adverse effects of these compounds have made it impossible to justify their long-term use for the disease. However, the experience with such drugs has been pivotal in efforts to prevent type 1 diabetes through immunotherapy[36].

In this section the results of several randomized trials of cyclosporine, azathioprine and corticosteroids for established type 1 diabetes will be briefly presented as well as their most important implications.

The first randomized, placebo-controlled, double-blind trial of cyclosporine for type 1 diabetes realized by a French multicentered group is worth noting[37]. In this study, 122 patients (age range 15–40 years) with a mean duration of symptomatic hyperglycemia of 10 weeks were randomized to receive cyclosporine or placebo. All patients were followed up for 6 months and 106 patients were followed for 9 months. Cyclosporine therapy led to higher rates of complete and partial remissions at 9 months and higher combined rates of partial remissions at 6 and 9 months. Within the cyclosporine group, complete remissions at 9 months were associated with blood cyclosporine levels ≥ 300 ng/ml during the first months of administration[36].

Another randomized, double-blind, placebo-controlled trial of cyclosporine for type 1 diabetes was performed in Canada and Europe[38]. In this study, 188 patients (aged between 10 and 35 years) were randomized within 14 weeks of symptom onset and 6 weeks of starting insulin treatment. Blinding was maintained for 1 year, during which period the subjects were assessed every 3 months for clinical response and insulin secretion by glucagon-stimulated C-peptide levels. Non-insulin-receiving remissions were more frequent in the cyclosporine group at 6 and 12 months. The cyclosporine group had higher mean glucagon-stimulated C-peptide at 90 days, which was maintained at 1 year, while the mean value in the placebo group fell progressively after 3 months. A strong interaction between the treatment group, duration of disease and non-insulin-receiving remission was shown by a *post hoc* subgroup analysis[36].

Two smaller randomized controlled trials of cyclosporine in recent-onset type 1 diabetes were completed in the USA[39,40]. In a Miami trial, 23 patients were randomized to cyclosporine or placebo for 1 year. Cyclosporine administration was associated with significantly higher meal-stimulated C-peptide levels through this time. In an open trial from Denver, 43 patients were randomized to receive cyclosporine for 4 months or no immunosuppression. No differences were seen between the two groups over 3 years in glycated hemoglobin (GHb) levels, remissions or C-peptide secretion[36].

A randomized double-blind, placebo-controlled trial of azathioprine for newly diagnosed type 1 diabetes was reported from Australia[41]. A group of 49 patients (age range 2–20 years) with a mean duration of symptomatic diabetes of 20 days were randomized and followed for 1 year. Complete remissions were not seen in either group; nor were significant differences found in mean GHb levels, insulin dosage or rates of partial remissions at 6 and 12 months. A significant increase in fasting C-peptide over the first 3 months occurred in the azathioprine group and was maintained to 6 months[36].

In a study from Gainesville (USA), 46 patients (age range 4–33 years) with symptomatic type 1 diabetes of up to 150 days were randomized to open therapy with azathioprine for 1 year plus corticosteroids (four doses of intravenous methylprednisone followed by a 10-week tapering course of prednisone) or no immunosuppression[42]. Although more patients receiving immunosuppression (10) than controls (2) discontinued insulin for at least 1 week over 12 months, this difference was not significant. After 1 year, three patients receiving immunosuppression had normal blood glucose and GHb without insulin treatment whereas all control patients were receiving insulin. *Post hoc* analyses demonstrated that better metabolic control and older age at entry were associated with improved metabolic status at 1 year among patients receiving immunosuppression[36].

Although the utilization of cyclosporine, azathioprine and corticosteroids in the treatment of the initial phases of type 1 diabetes is associated with major risks, the clinical trials of these agents have been very important in the continuing efforts to discover safe and efficient immunotherapy for diabetes. Mahon and Dupre summarized the principal scientific benefits of these studies.

1. They have brought definite proof that an immune-mediated process determines beta-cell loss in human type 1 diabetes. All other observations before these trials could only yield circumstantial evidence for this conclusion.
2. Another basic observation is that T lymphocytes play a central role in human beta-cell loss. Humoral mechanisms are not of primary significance in the pathogenesis of this process.
3. The experience with the above-mentioned drugs drew attention to the importance of accounting for insulin action when assessing clinical efficiency in future preventive trials.

4. It has been conclusively demonstrated that a cause–effect relationship between improved endogenous insulin secretion and improved glycemic control exists. This finding is very important for the conception of future strategies for the primary and secondary prevention of type 1 diabetes.
5. It has also been demonstrated that the intensity of beta-cell destruction may fluctuate[36].

These findings stimulate an optimistic approach to the problems of the prevention of type 1 diabetes and its consequences.

4.4   INSULIN

The capacity to identify subjects at risk for type 1 diabetes makes the search for new immune-based intervention strategies during the prodromal period (with a view to preventing or delaying clinical onset of the disease) a major goal. Furthermore, there is now general agreement that immunologic intervention may be most efficient if started early in the disease process. Increasing interest is being expressed in prophylactic insulin therapy as antigen-specific immuno-regulatory therapy for secondary level prevention[43,44].

It is known that insulin is the only target autoantigen identified in human type 1 diabetes which is exclusively beta-cell specific, whereas glutamic acid decarboxylase and tyrosine phosphatase IA2/ICA 512 are also expressed in the pancreas and the brain[45,46]. Insulin auto-antibodies can be detected years before clinical manifestation of the disease[47]. Anti-insulin autoimmunity can also be demonstrated at the T-lymphocyte level[48]. More recently, insulin-specific T-lymphocyte lines and clones were isolated from islet-infiltrating lymphocytes of NOD mice. Proliferative tests showed that these insulin-specific T-lymphocyte clones responded vigorously to a peptide of the insulin B-chain "B9-B23"[49]. There could also be a direct regenerative effect on antiapoptotic or proregenerative beta cells[50].

4.4.1   Insulin Preventive Therapy in Animal Models

This was mentioned briefly in Chapter 3. The effects of prophylactic insulin treatment seem to depend on a variety of factors related to the antigenicity of the antigen fragment, the antigen dosage, the initiation and duration of therapy, the route of application and the carrier by which insulin is delivered. Three different approaches have been utilized in animal models: (1) daily subcutaneous administration of insulin; (2) daily oral administration of insulin; (3) intermittent immunization with insulin and its metabolically inactive A- and B-chains in incomplete Freund's adjuvant[43].

Insulin delivery to BB rats starting at 35–40 days of age and continuing till 120 days, by implantable insulinomas or mini-pumps, significantly decreased the incidence of diabetes as well as the incidence of insulitis[51]. The decrease of insulitis shows an effect on the basic disease process, separate from any simple metabolic action[52]. In another study, BB rats were treated with ultralente insulin between 40 and 142 days of age; a reduction of diabetes and insulitis was observed[53]. The same effect has been seen with insulin given as a subcutaneous injection five times a week from 35 to 120 days of age[54]. At our Animal Diabetes Department in Bucharest, we obtained similar results with daily injections of MC lente insulin (Novo Nordisk) or Iletin (Eli Lilly) and also by subcutaneous introduction of fragments of insulinic implants—Linplant, Linshin, Canada (unpublished observations).

Comparable results were obtained in NOD mice given daily protamine zinc insulin by injection at weaning: diabetes and insulitis were decreased[55]. As in the BB rats, insulin administration also protected NOD mice from adoptive transfer of diabetes[56]. Other authors analyzed the effects of parenteral insulin by using an "immunization" schedule, injecting insulin with incomplete Freund's adjuvant at intervals of 4–8 weeks to a total of four injections. Insulin given in this way would have very little metabolic effect and was very efficient in preventing diabetes and insulitis. Insulin B-chain given in the same manner was also effective, although the insulin A-chain and insulin diluent were not efficient[57]. A recombinant monomeric human insulin analog, which does not bind to the insulin receptor as a consequence of an alteration of a single amino acid at position 25 of the B-chain, was shown to be as effective at diabetes prevention as was intact insulin. In contrast to native insulin, the insulin analog did not cause hypoglycemia after subcutaneous injection[58].

The data obtained from animal studies thus indicate that prophylactic insulin administration may offer protection from diabetes, although that protection is not complete because a variety of factors seem to determine its extent[43]. One explanation for the beneficial effect, is "beta-cell rest" which results from a metabolic effect of insulin on the beta cell. If the metabolic activity of the beta cell is decreased, it may be less susceptible to specific immune damage[52,59]. Another explanation appears to be connected to the immune modulatory effects of insulin as an important beta-cell antigen, since immunizing doses and B-chains are also effective[43,50,52]. This final explanation will be discussed in greater detail in Section 4.5.

4.4.2   Insulin Preventive Therapy in Human Subjects

In this section, we will discuss those trials based on the utilization of parenteral insulin (Table 4.1).

Table 4.1. Human pilot trials for prophylactic insulin therapy (results obtained by 1995)

Name of trial	Design	Insulin route	Diabetes incidence in treated subjects	Diabetes incidence in controls
Joslin Pilot (USA)	Open, controlled, non-randomized	Intravenous + subcutaneous	2/5	7/7
Schwabing Insulin Prophylaxis (SIP) Pilot (Germany)	Open, controlled, randomized	Intravenous + subcutaneous	2/7	3/6
Spain	Open, controlled, randomized	Subcutaneous	1/5	2/5
Boston– Denver (USA)	Placebo-controlled, randomized	Intravenous Subcutaneous Intranvenous + Subcutaneous	3/7 0/6 0/3	1/1

Adapted from reference 43

Insulin prophylaxis in human pre-type 1 diabetes was used for the first time at the Joslin's Diabetes Center, USA[60]. A group of 12 first-degree relatives, aged between 7 and 40 years, who were identified to be at high risk for the development of type 1 diabetes using an assessment derived from the "Joslin dual-parameter model" (that is >72% risk of diabetes within 3 years of follow up) were eligible for the prevention protocol. Of these, five accepted the administration of insulin and seven refused. All participants were required to have a normal result on OGTT and to express ICA as well as to have IAA and/or a low first-phase insulin secretion determined using an IVGTT. The results were essentially as follows: two of five children treated with 5-day courses of intravenous insulin every 9 months, followed by daily low-dose subcutaneous insulin, developed diabetes, compared with all seven untreated controls. The results showed that the insulin regimen was practical and that there was minimal hypoglycemia, which resolved spontaneously or with the use of simple measures. The subjects received an average of 0.22 units of insulin per day. The authors chose this minimal dosage with the aim of changing the subjects' lifestyles as little as possible—with the exception of injections before breakfast and before bed[52].

With regard to the subjects that developed diabetes, several things must be said: two of the treated subjects developed diabetes, though onset was later than predicted. These two had the highest diabetes risk—and in fact their "predicted time" to diabetes was negative with the model used. The seven subjects who declined treatment all developed diabetes within 2.2 years[52,60].

Entry into the pilot study was stopped after the initial 12 subjects and a randomized controlled trial of parenteral insulin was begun. This study has since evolved into a multicenter NIH-sponsored trial designated the Diabetes Prevention Trial—Type 1 or DTP-1[52].

As can be seen from Table 4.1, other randomized pilot studies have been initiated in Germany, Spain and the USA in order to verify the efficacy of different treatment regimens in prevention of clinical type 1 diabetes in high-risk relatives. All trials used similar entry criteria and included relatives that had been predicted to have at least 75% probability of developing the disease within 5 years. Risk staging of non-diabetic first-degree relatives with normal OGTTs was based on ICA-positivity ($> 20\,$JDF units) and low first-phase insulin release ($1 + 3$-minute insulin $< 65\,$mU/l) for both the German and Spanish trials. Risk factors staging for the Boston–Denver trial were considered on the dual parameter model of prediction[43].

The aim of the Spanish open, controlled, pilot trial was to evaluate the effect of subcutaneous insulin administration on the natural course of the prediabetic state[61]. The study included 10 high-risk relatives of whom five accepted insulin treatment with 0.1 U of NPH insulin/kg and five were used as controls. Only one of five treated individuals developed clinical diabetes after 20 months of treatment whereas two of the controls developed the disease, at 4 and 18 months of follow up respectively. In the insulin-treated group, ICA titer decreased in two subjects and was negative in three; in the control group an increase of the ICA titers was found (3/5).

In 1992, in Boston and Denver (USA) a randomized placebo-controlled pilot trial was initiated in order to continue the study of subcutaneous (SC) plus intravenous (IV) insulin administration and extended with different treatment arms including SC insulin alone, IV insulin alone and IV placebo. Until May 1995, three of seven subjects on the IV arm, but none of six subjects on the SC arm had developed clinical diabetes (CS Eisenbarth, personal communication; cited in reference 43).

EPP-SCIT is a randomized trial concerning children at very high risk initiated in Europe[50].

In a recent paper the results of the Schwabing Insulin Prophylaxis (SIP) Pilot Trial started in Germany in 1990 were published[62]. This was a randomized, controlled pilot study designed to determine whether insulin treatment can prevent or delay the clinical onset of type 1 diabetes in high-risk first-degree relatives of the patients. In this trial, the first-degree relatives of type 1 diabetics, aged 4 years or more with ICA titers greater than 20 JDF units, a reduced first-phase insulin response to an IV tolerance test less than the fifth centile and a normal OGTT were recruited. Between January 1989 and October 1995, 1736 candidates were screened for ICA. The authors identified 64 cases (3.7%) with ICA levels greater than 20 JDF units. Of the ICA-positive relatives, 17 (27%) had a low first-phase insulin response and were eligible for enrolment. Of these, 14 agreed to participate—seven were randomized to the treatment group and seven to the control group. In the treatment group, human insulin was given intravenously by continuous infusion for 7 days followed by daily subcutaneous administration for 6 months. Insulin infusions were repeated every 12 months.

The main results were that in the treatment group, three of the seven subjects (follow up from time of eligibility: 2.3–7.1 years) and in the control group six of the seven untreated subjects (1.7–7.1 years) developed the disease. Life table analysis showed that clinical onset of type 1 diabetes was delayed in insulin-treated subjects (mean ± SEM diabetes-free survival: 5.0 ± 0.9 years vs 2.3 ± 0.7 years, $p < 0.03$). Insulin levels after IV glucose increased in the first year of therapy. Titers of ICA, antibodies to GAD and tyrosine phosphatase-like protein IA2 were unchanged. These results suggest that insulin prophylaxis can delay the onset of clinical diabetes in high-risk relatives. The authors consider that the data obtained are encouraging in view of

- the ongoing American Diabetes Prevention Trial, which is currently testing the effect of parenteral insulin in a large nationwide study, and
- the initiation of pilot trials to determine whether new antigen-specific intervention is more effective in delaying the clinical onset of type 1 diabetes.

The authors do not shrink from recognizing that the protocols of the SIP Pilot Trial and of similar studies have several significant disadvantages, amongst which are admission to hospital for treatment and the difficulties of IVGTT. For this reason, they propose that future intervention trials and risk evaluations be based only on elevated antibodies. Also, treatment protocols should be considered that are more convenient for high-risk individuals in the general population[62].

The DPT-1 is a nationwide study designed to determine whether insulin-based procedures can prevent or delay overt type 1 diabetes in relatives found to be at high risk[63,64]. Parenteral insulin is used in relatives with $> 50\%$ projected 5-year risk; oral insulin is used in relatives with 26–50% projected 5-year risk. Screening of relatives of individuals with type 1 diabetes began in February 1994. Randomization began in December 1995 for the parenteral protocol and in September 1996 for the oral protocol. Of the 40 381 samples analyzed for ICA by November 30, 1996, 1391 were positive. Staging for risk was carried out in 937 individuals, 259 of whom had low first-phase insulin response to IVGTT. Of the subjects who were completely staged for risk categorization, 141 were eligible for the parenteral study and of these 131 (92.9% of the eligible) were randomized to the parenteral study. The oral study had 28 eligible subjects and 26 (92.9%) of these were randomized. Overall enrollment rates were 74.4% of those projected for the parenteral study and 89.7% of those projected for the oral study at the time of publication[64,65].

The DPT-1 trial aims to screen a total of 60 000–80 000 first-degree relatives of patients with type 1 diabetes. The subjects of the intervention will be followed over a period of 5–6 years. The investigators believe that this trial will serve as a prototype for any future intervention studies, whether refinements of insulin therapy are being explored or new methods are being tried[52].

After the first preventive trials with parenteral insulin, Füchtenbush and Ziegler concluded that the combination of intravenous and subcutaneous insulin seems to be most efficient followed by subcutaneous insulin alone[43]. Intravenous insulin alone and temporary subcutaneous insulin in combination with intravenous insulin appear to be less effective[43].

4.5   ORAL ANTIGEN TOLERIZATION

In this section one of the most interesting and encouraging methods to date of obtaining some major progress in type 1 diabetes prevention will be presented.

4.5.1   Scientific Background

As has been underlined by Weiner[66], the goal of treatment for autoimmnune disorders is to specifically suppress the autoreactive immune processes without affecting the rest of the immune system. Oral tolerance represents the exogenous administration of antigen to the peripheral immune system via the intestine. Basically, there are three mechanisms to explain antigen-driven tolerance: clonal deletion, clonal anergy and active suppression. A number of studies have shown that one of the primary mechanisms associated with oral tolerance is active suppression. Later, clonal anergy and in some instances clonal deletion, may occur. The type of tolerance obtained is correlated with the antigen dose[66].

The gut-associated lymphoid tissue (GALT) comprises lymphoid nodules termed Peyer's patches, villi containing epithelial cells and intraepithelial lymphocytes and lymphocytes scattered throughout the lamina propria[67]. In the Peyer's patches regulatory cells are generated which mediate the active suppression component of oral tolerance. In addition, it has been suggested that Th2-type responses may be preferentially generated in Peyer's patches[66,68]. Intraepithelial lymphocytes are oligoclonal, activated and cytolytic but proliferate poorly. Lamina propria lymphocytes are found diffusely interspersed in the lamina propria, with a $CD4^+/CD8^+$ cell ratio closely resembling those of the Peyer's patches and peripheral blood[67].

As has already been mentioned, a very important factor that determines which form of peripheral tolerance develops following oral administration of antigen is the quantity of antigen fed. Low doses of antigen favor the generation of active suppression or regulatory cell-driven tolerance whereas high doses favor anergy-driven tolerance. These two forms are not mutually exclusive; however, they are distinct and the use of oral tolerance to treat autoimmune diseases such as type 1 diabetes is critically dependent on which is triggered[66].

Although dietary antigens are degraded by the time they reach the small intestine, investigations in humans and rodents have shown that degradation is partial and that some intact antigen is also absorbed[69].

A series of research projects on oral tolerance in autoimmune models have found active suppression to be a primary mechanism and have identified regulatory cells, generated following oral toler-ance, which act by secreting antigen-non-specific down regulatory cytokines[70]. It has also become clear that in human autoimmune diseases such as multiple sclerosis and type 1 diabetes there is, most probably, reactivity to multiple autoantigens from the target tissue, even if the disease was initiated by a single antigen. The mechanism of bystander suppression following oral tolerance obviates this major conceptual problem. Bystander suppression was first demonstrated *in vitro* and then *in vivo*. It is specific to the fed antigen and is transfer-able[66,71].

The immaturity of the immunoregulatory network associated with oral tolerance and sensitization to autoantigens via the gut in the neonatal period may contribute to the pathogenesis of autoimmune diseases. This hypothesis is in concordance with studies in which it is demonstrated that the exposure to cows' milk during early infancy determines, in individuals genetically susceptible to type 1 diabetes, the development of anti-BSA antibodies that cross-react with a beta-cell surface protein[72].

The treatment of animals with IFN-γ abrogated oral tolerance, as measured by antibody responses to orally administered BSA[73]. A series of other factors could also intervene in the modulation of oral tolerance[66].

The process of antigen presentation within the gut is very important for the generation of active suppression. There are several cells capable of antigen presentation in the gut-associated lymphoid tissue, including macrophages and dendritic cells in the Peyer's patches and lamina propria, B lymphocytes and epithelial cells. MHC class II is constitutively expressed on the small intestine epithelium[74]. It is possible that the cells mentioned above preferentially stimulate Th2-type responses because of the gut environment, specific properties of the antigen-presenting cells or different costimulatory signals[66].

Numerous papers have shown that orally administered autoantigens can suppress experimental models of autoimmunity. Thus, the oral administration of myelin basic protein from the guinea-pig to suppress experimental autoimmine encephalomyelitis (EAE) was first shown in the Lewis rat model[75]. The suppression of collagen-induced arthritis by feeding collagen type II has been demonstrated[76]. Experimental allergic uveitis, experimental autoimmune myasthenia gravis, thyroiditis and transplantation represent other conclusive examples[66].

In human subjects, there have been some interesting studies in multiple sclerosis (using bovine myelin), rheumatoid arthritis (with oral collagen), uveitis and other conditions.

Bearing in mind the results obtained in animal models of autoimmunity and the initial studies in humans, it appears that orally administered autoantigens may find a place in the treatment of human organ-specific autoimmune diseases. Such treatment would have the advantages of being orally administered, non-toxic and antigen specific[66].

4.5.2   Studies in Animal Diabetes

This section will begin with several observations on the activity of orally administered insulin. This has no hypoglycemic effects because it is broken down by gastric and pancreatic proteases. Over the years it has been thought that the situation could be changed with the aid of substances like alcohol, saponins, resorcinol or quinine but most of these findings were not confirmed and are now of historical interest only[77,78].

Studies related to duodenal, jejunal or ileal administration of insulin deserve special attention. The investigations carried out in rabbits showed that: (a) intrajejunal administration of 20 U/kg insulin did not produce a modification of blood glucose during an observation period of 3 hours; (b) intraduodenal or intrajejunal administration of 50 U/kg insulin did not modify blood glucose during a period of 7 hours; (c) intrajejunal administration of 150 U/kg insulin produced a hypoglycemic effect approximately equivalent to that produced by 0.2 U/kg injected intramuscularly[79]. A treatment of alloxan-diabetic rats with intrajejunal administration of 250–500 U/kg insulin in water-in-oil-in-water emulsions produced hypoglycemic effects similar to those obtained with intramuscular regular insulin at doses of 1–2 U/kg[80].

The results of other studies show that insulin can pass through the intestinal wall of the infant rat, the infant mouse, the newborn pig and the newborn calf[81,82]. Similarly, an increased passage of insulin through the intestinal wall has been demonstrated when pancreatic enzymes are absent or have been inactivated in the gut wall[83]. In these experiments, doses of 40–250 U/kg insulin were required to produce a metabolic effect.

In another study, 100 U/kg insulin was injected directly into the upper jejunum, of a human diabetic subject who had been pancreatectomized and in a healthy 46-year-old man[84]. In the pancreatectomized and diabetic subject, a moderate reduction in glycemia has been observed (from 300 to 200 mg%) after the third hour following treatment. On the contrary, no change in blood glucose levels was noted in the healthy subject receiving a total of 6400 U insulin during a follow-up period of 8 hours.

From these works, the following conclusions can be made:

1. Oral administration of insulin does not produce metabolic effects because of the breakdown of the hormone by gastric and pancreatic preoteases.
2. Hypoglycemic effects have been observed in several animal models when insulin is directly injected into the duodenum or the upper jejunum, but at doses higher than 50 U/kg.
3. In several animal and human models, the hypoglycemic effect of oral insulin is increased during the first days of life as well as in subjects with inactivated or absent pancreatic enzymes (A. Falorni, personal communication).

Alternatively, insulin may induce specific enzyme tolerance independent of its effects on islet beta-cell metabolic activity[43]. This idea is supported by the results published by Zhang *et al.*, who set out to examine whether oral administration of insulin is efficient in influencing the natural course of diabetes in NOD mice[85]. They showed that animals fed with 1 mg of oral porcine insulin per week from the age of 5 weeks up to the age of 1 year subsequently had a decreased incidence of diabetes (20% compared with 43% of control litter at 1 year of age) and reduced degrees of insulitis. In addition, protection appeared to be disease specific because oral insulin did not prevent the development of EAE in SJL mice. As expected, oral insulin did not change blood glucose levels, ruling out protection by "islet beta-cell rest". The dose of the antigen seemed crucial to the efficacy of tolerance induction: doses of less than 1 mg and those of 5 mg were not protective.

Muir *et al.* could not find a reduction of the final incidence of diabetes in NOD mice fed with oral insulin (0.5 mg every second day, 1 mg every second week), but did demonstrate a delay of the onset of the disease by 6–12 weeks[86]. These differences may have been due to different dosing intervals or a difference between strains of the NOD mice[43].

It has been shown that acceleration of diabetes was suppressed by splenocytes from NOD mice fed 1 mg of oral insulin, but not by splenocytes from NOD mice fed with buffer or myelin basic protein[85]. Another study reported that T lymphocytes from the spleens of diabetic female NOD donors, co-infused with the same number of splenic T lymphocytes from insulin-fed animals into irradiated recipient mice, decreased the diabetes transfer rate by 50%[87]. Therefore, not only the amount of insulin but also the duration of treatment seems to be crucial for effective protection as animals fed for 15 days instead of 30 days lost the capacity for adoptive protection[43].

The ability to suppress insulitis by administering the B-chain of insulin, peptides of the B-chain or GAD has been demonstrated.

Immunohistochemical studies were performed on animals fed porcine insulin over a 5-week period. There was an increase in IL-4, IL-10, PGE and TGF-β in the islets of insulin-fed animals and a decrease of IFN-γ, TNF-α and IL-2[88]. These results suggest that a Th2-type response is being generated in association with the ameliorating effects of oral insulin[66].

It has also been shown that oral administration of insulin can induce the presence of regulatory T cells in the pancreas and the corresponding draining lymph nodes, initiate the secretion of IL-4 in this microenvironment sufficiently to suppress the activity of Th1 autoreactive T-cell clones and ultimately provide protection against autoimmune diabetes[89].

From what has been expressed so far, it appears that the effect of oral insulin is quite limited and that the disease suppression is limited to a narrow dose range. A group of German authors tried to improve the outcome of suboptimal insulin dosing by using a bacterial adjuvant[90]. Mice treated with a suboptimal dose of oral insulin showed no modification of diabetes incidence although a shift from Th1 towards Th2 cytokine expression was detected in inflamed islets. Significant suppression of diabetes development was demonstrated in NOD mice receiving both insulin and the bacterial preparation designated OM-89. This is a protein extract from *Escherichia coli* with non-specific immunostimulatory properties. Potentiation of the effect of oral insulin by the bacterial adjuvant was associated with upregulation of IL-4 Th2 cells in infiltrated islets and sustained local IL-2 gene expression. Analyses of cytokine expression in the gut using reverse transcriptase polymerase chain reaction showed a clear deviation to Th2-type reactivity and downregulation of inducible nitric oxide synthase (iNOS) expression by the bacterial adjuvant alone but not by insulin alone. Since macrophages are the primary target cells of adjuvant action, the authors tested its effect on mouse macrophages *in vitro*. Treatment with OM-89 induced transient release of TNF-α and nitrite but rendered macrophages refractory to restimulation by the potent macrophage activator lipopolysaccharide.

The authors of the study arrived at the conclusion that the protective effect of oral insulin on the progression of insulitis and the development of overt diabetes in NOD mice can be potentiated by pretreatment with the bacterial adjuvant OM-89. The effect correlated with enhanced Th2 cytokine and decreased iNOS gene expression, probably as a consequence of local downregulation of proinflammatory Th1-type mediators by exposure to the adjuvant[90].

In order to potentiate oral tolerance against autoimmune diabetes, insulin conjugated to the cholera toxin B (CTB) subunit was administered orally to NOD mice[91]. A single feeding of 100 μg of CTB-insulin to 10-week-old females reduced the incidence of clinical diabetes at 21 weeks of age. Lower concentrations of CTB-insulin were able to delay diabetes onset but did not significantly decrease the final diabetes incidence. During co-transfer experiments, T cells from the spleens of 8-week-old females fed one week before with 10 μg of CTB-insulin were able to reduce the capability of the diabetogenic T cells to transfer diabetes in irradiated NOD male recipients. These protective effects were associated with a significant increase in the percentage of normal islets and islets with peri-insulitis as well as a significant reduction in the number of severely infiltrated islets. Preliminary co-transfer experiments using NOD mice congenic at the Thy-1 locus indicated that T cells from CTB-insulin fed animals were not present in the thymuses of recipient mice 15 days after cell transfer and were increased in the pancreatic lymph nodes in these animals compared with mice reconstituted with diabetogenic T cells and T lymphocytes from CTB-fed animals, which suggested a local mechanism of regulation. The authors believe that this new strategy of tolerance induction may have important consequences for prevention and treatment of autoimmune diabetes[91].

Sobel *et al.* have shown that CTB administration prevents the development of diabetes in NOD mice by inhibiting immune destruction of the islets[92]. The islet-sparing activity appears mediated, at least in part, by the induction of regulatory cells and, in turn, suppression of anti-islet effector cells, which is not associated with generalized immunosuppression or T- or B-cell depletion[92].

No protective effect of oral insulin in the BB rat was observed[93]. A new study was recently carried out by Bellman *et al.*[94]. Bearing in mind the positive outcome of the previous studies in NOD mice, BB rats received insulin in combination with a bacterial adjuvant. Porcine insulin was given orally twice a week from 35 to 100 days of age; the *Escherichia coli* preparation OM-89 was fed on alternate days. Other groups of animals received vehicle, the bacterial adjuvant or insulin alone. Both insulin-containing oral dosing regimens induced a transient, insignificant, delay in diabetes onset. Insulin alone, however, did not reduce the final diabetes incidence. Oral dosing with insulin plus adjuvant exacerbated the development of disease, as judged by the decreased survival rate compared with the insulin treated group. Intra-islet infiltration is also increased compared with the insulin or vehicle-treated groups. This effect correlated with enhanced IFN-γ and decreased IL-10 gene expression in the gut, suggesting a shift towards proinflammatory Th1 reactivity. Although treatment with adjuvant alone also increased the degree of insulitis, enhanced incidence of diabetes and a shift in cytokine expression was seen only in the group receiving insulin plus adjuvant.

The authors consider that the gut immune system of BB rats is biased towards inflammatory Th1 reactivity, in contrast with NOD mice, and exhibits impaired oral tolerance. The results further underline an important role for the gut in the pathogenesis of type 1 diabetes. The treatment with a bacterial adjuvant and oral insulin in BB rats may modify the gut immunoregulatory state such that disease-promoting rather than protective immune responses are produced[94].

4.5.3   Studies in Human Diabetes

As has already been mentioned, DPT-1 includes two forms of insulin intervention: parenteral and oral[66,95]. The protocol involving oral administration of insulin is destined for "intermediate-risk" (25–50% over 5 years) subjects. The oral trial is placebo controlled and double masked. Relatives aged 3–45 years positive for both ICA (≥ 10 JDF units) and IAA (≥ 80 nU/ml), not HLA-DQA1*0102 or DQB1*0602, whose IVGTT-insulin $\Sigma(1' + 3')$ do not meet "high risk" criteria and who have normal glucose tolerance, will be eligible. The goal is to randomize 500 subjects in approximately equal numbers to active or placebo therapy. Eligible subjects will be recruited from

60–80 000 relatives to be screened for ICA over a 4-year period. Randomized subjects will receive either 7.5 mg/day of oral recombinant human insulin crystals or placebo taken as a capsule or sprinkled on food. Patients will be verified by OGTT (baseline and every 6 months) to exclude development of type 1 diabetes and evaluate pancreatic beta-cell function. IVGTTs (baseline and every 12 months) and mixed meal tolerance testing (baseline and every 36 months) will further assess beta-cell function. The results of the study will be analyzed sequentially and evaluated by an external monitoring group. All statistical analyses of differences between treatment groups will include all subjects randomized into the trial, regardless of adherence. Interim analyses will also include monitoring for patient safety, protocol compliance and data quality[95]. The oral arm of DPT-1 began in September 1996. From time to time, the authors informed the international scientific community of the progress of its principal aspects[33,65].

The DIOR trial initiated in France is related to recently diabetic children and adults[50].

4.5.4 European Diabetes Oral Tolerance Study

The initiative for this study was taken by the Dipartimento di Medicina Interna e Scienze Endocrine e Metaboliche (DIMISEM), University of Perugia, Italy, led by Professor Paolo Brunetti. Dr Alberto Falorni works in the capacity of principal investigator. In his application for a JDFI Research Grant (January 1997), Dr Falorni defined the project as a European multicenter, double-blind/triple antigen-specific autoantibody-positive, HLA-DQB1*0602-negative trial of first-degree relatives of IDDM patients. The specific aims of this project are:

1. To test the hypothesis that residual insulin production can be preserved in double/triple autoantibody-positive first-degree relatives of type 1 patients by oral insulin tolerization.
2. To test the hypothesis that clinical type 1 diabetes can be effectively prevented in double/triple autoantibody-positive first-degree relatives of type 1 diabetic patients by oral insulin tolerization.

3. To evaluate the efficacy of oral insulin tolerization in subjects with either normal or reduced first-phase insulin response after metabolic stimulation.
4. To evaluate the predictive value of antigen-specific type 1 diabetes-associated autoantibodies in first-degree relatives of patients from high (Sweden) and medium/low (Italy/Greece) risk populations.
5. To test the hypothesis that autoantibody screening of first-degree relatives can be useful for an early diagnosis of previously unknown diabetes mellitus.

Initially, it was estimated that a total number of 6000 first-degree relatives would suffice for the identification of the 120 at-risk subjects required for the study. All the serum samples from first-degree relatives will be tested for the presence of antibodies against GAD65 and/or IA-2/ICA512 using radioimmunoassays with recombinant human antigen[96]. In addition, the levels of IAA (in a competitive radioimmunoassay) and ICA (in an indirect immuno-fluorescence assay) will be evaluated[97,98]. All individuals found positive for at least two antigen-specific autoantibodies will be considered for the trial.

Before entering the prevention trial, double/triple autoantibody-positive, non-diabetic subjects will be tested for the presence or absence of the HLA-DQB*0602 allele. The positive subjects will be excluded. In all the subjects entering the trial, an IVGTT would be performed and the FPIR $(1' + 3')$ would be evaluated[99]. The results of the IVGTT would not be used as an inclusion criterion but only for statistical purposes. Each at-risk first-degree relative who agrees to enter the trial would be randomly assigned to one of the two study groups (either oral insulin or placebo). Adequate oral slow-releasing insulin and placebo preparations will be made available by Novo Nordisk A/S. Treated subjects would be followed up for a minimum period of 5 years.

Several European diabetes centers (from Italy, Sweden, Germany, Greece, Romania) agreed to participate in this project from its earliest stages. The participation of additional European centers would be encouraged.

The First Meeting of the European Study Group on Immunoprevention of IDDM by Oral Insulin Tolerization that took place in Perugia, Italy on 13 September 1997 was an important moment for the completion of the initially proposed protocol and also for the clarification of some controversial aspects of the project. In addition to a strong team from DIMISEM (Professor Paolo Brunetti, Dr Alberto Falorni, Dr Filippo Calcinaro, Professor Massimo Massi-Benedetti, Professor Fausto Santeusanio and Dr Georgia Kassi), other personalities from different countries made valuable contributions to this meeting. These include Professor Åke Lernmark (Seattle, USA), Dr Jacob Petersen (Zymogenetics, Seattle, USA), Dr Patrizio Pezzotti (Rome, Italy), Professor Bengt Persson (Stockholm, Sweden), Professor G. Brabant (Hannover, Germany), Dr Thomas Dryberg (Novo Nordisk, Copenhagen, Denmark) and representatives of the countries mentioned above.

After the discussions held in Perugia, the protocol for the identification of subjects at high risk for type 1 diabetes remained basically unchanged: 5–39-year-old first-degree relatives of the patients will be studied for the presence and levels of GAD65Ab and/or IA2Ab. In autoantibody-positive subjects, levels of IAA and ICA will then be evaluated. Based on the observations of Professor Lernmark, the presence of the protective HLA-DQB1*0602 haplotype would be used as an exclusion criterion only for subjects younger than 15 years.

The major discussions and decisions were related to the cholera toxin subunit B. I have already related some of the promising results obtained from NOD mice using CTB-insulin conjugates[91,92]. A series of studies carried out at Zymogenetics, Seattle, USA (J. Petersen, personal communication) demonstrated that feeding NOD mice weekly with a mixture of CTB and insulin brought about the suppression of clinical diabetes to an extent similar to that observed when using the CTB conjugate. Thus, the use of CTB potentiated oral tolerance to insulin in such a way that a 10-fold lower dose of insulin was sufficient to prevent diabetes. Also, a CTB-insulin mixture was as effective as the CTB-insulin conjugate in reducing islet inflammatory infiltrate. In Table 4.2 the different procedures for oral insulin tolerization in NOD mice are summarized. This kind of study on the NOD mouse represents a scientific background for the use of a mixture of insulin and CTB in clinical trials of type 1 diabetes prevention by oral tolerization.

Finally, it was decided that recombinant CTB with proven benefits in oral administration be used[100,101]. To date, there is no knowledge of side-effects of oral therapy with recombinant CTB.

Table 4.2. Different procedures for oral insulin tolerization in NOD mice

Type of procedure	Essential reference
Insulin alone	Zhang et al.[85]
Insulin and OM-89 (a protein extract of E. coli)	Hartmann et al.[90]
CTB*-insulin conjugates	Bergerot et al.[91]
Mixture of insulin and CTB	Petersen (personal communication, 1997)

*Cholera toxin B

At the time of the writing, the screening of first-degree relatives of type 1 diabetes subjects is under way.

4.6 FUTURE DIRECTIONS

The perspectives for the prevention of type 1 diabetes mellitus are many and very interesting. Table 4.3 attempts a systematic presentation (after Skyler and Marks[102]). The authors feel that the final goal is development of vaccine preparations that are capable of stimulating the generation of vigorous responses without triggering side-effects. Their prediction is that insulin, insulin B-chain or a fragment peptide of insulin B-chain will be used in large vaccination programs to prevent type 1 diabetes.

In this chapter, I have highlighted the use of prophylactic insulin via the parenteral and oral routes. The main human trials, still in process, are based on these two paths. It is now time to mention the use of nasal insulin.

Harrison et al. began with the idea that cellular immune hypo-responsiveness can be induced by the presentation of soluble protein antigens to mucosal surfaces[103]. When they administered insulin aerosol to NOD mice even after the onset of subclinical disease, pancreatic islet pathology and diabetes incidence were significantly decreased. Insulin-treated mice had increased circulating antibodies to insulin and reduced splenic T-cell proliferation to the major epitope, insulin B-chain amino acids 9–23, associated with increased IL-4 and especially IL-10 production as well as reduced proliferation to GAD.

Table 4.3. Future directions in prevention of type 1 diabetes

---

Peptide-mediated immunotherapy:
 Peptide immunization
 Peptides as specific T-cell receptor (TCR) antagonists
 Induction of anergy
 HLA-derived peptides
 Superantigen-based vaccines
Insulin and insulin peptides for peptide-mediated immunotherapy:
 Parenteral insulin
 Insulin vaccination
 Oral insulin
 Nasal insulin
Milk-protein-based immunotherapy
Immune system stimulation:
 Immunostimulant vaccines
 Linomide
Monoclonal antibody immunomodulation
Cytokine manipulation
T-cell vaccination
Tolerance induction
Prospects for gene therapy

Adapted from reference 102

The ability of splenocytes from insulin-treated mice to suppress adoptive transfer of diabetes by diabetogenic T cells shown to be due to small numbers of CD8$\gamma\delta$ T cells. These cells also inhibit cyclophosphamide-accelerated diabetes and may be responsible for regulating the natural history of islet autoimmunity in NOD mice. Induction of regulatory CD8$\gamma\delta$ T cells by aerosol insulin has implications for the prevention of human type 1 diabetes. The value of using intranasal insulin in humans has been verified by Harrison *et al.* in a double-blind, placebo-controlled, cross-over designed trial, commenced in Melbourne, Australia in June 1996. The subjects who began treatment are being tested monthly for autoantibodies (IAA, GAD, IA-2) and T-cell proliferative and cytokine (IFN-γ, IL-10, IL-5, TNF-α) responses to the relevent antigens. This study was completed at the end of 1998[33].

Many of the ideas put forward by researchers are daring and valuable. In principle, these must be confirmed through carefully designed, randomized, controlled trials[102]. Their organization requires not only scientific competence and energy but also significant financial support[33].

REFERENCES

1. Tuomilehto J, Wolf E. Primary prevention of diabetes mellitus. *Diabetes Care* 1987; **10**: 238–248.
2. Tuomilehto J, Tuomilehto-Wolf E, Zimmet P, Alberti KGMM, Knowler WC. Primary Prevention of Diabetes Mellitus. In Alberti KGMM, Zimmet P, DeFronzo RA, Keen H (eds). *International Textbook of Diabetes Mellitus*, 2nd edn. Chichester: Wiley, 1997; 1799–1827.
3. England WL, Roberts SD. Immunisation to prevent insulin-dependent diabetes mellitus? The economics of genetic screening and vaccination for diabetes. *Ann Intern Med* 1981; **94**: 395–400.
4. Saukkonen T, Virtanen SM, Karppinen M *et al.* and the Childhood Diabetes in Finland Study Group. Significance of cow's milk protein antibodies as risk factor for childhood IDDM: interactions with dietary cow's milk intake and HLA-DQB1 genotype. *Diabetologia* 1998; **41**: 72–78.
5. Ellis TM, Ottendorfer E, Jodoin E *et al.* Cellular immune responses to β casein: elevated in, but not specific for individuals with Type I diabetes mellitus. *Diabetologia* 1998; **41**: 731–735.
6. Åkerblom HK, Savilahti E, Saukkonen TT *et al.* The case for elimination of cow's milk in early infancy in the prevention of type 1 diabetes: the Finnish experience. *Diabetes Metab Rev* 1993; **9**: 269–278.
7. Pardini VC, Vieira JGH, Miranda W, Ferreira SRC, Velho G, Russo EMK. Antibodies to bovine serum albumin in Brazilian children and young adults with IDDM. *Diabetes Care* 1996; **19**: 126–129.
8. Åkerblom HK, Knip M. Prevention of IDDM: strategies based on new observations of molecular pathogenesis. *Diabetologia* 1997; **40**: 743–748.
9. Karges W, Hammond-McKibben D, Cheung RK *et al.* Immunological aspects of nutritional diabetes prevention in NOD mice: a pilot study for the cow's milk-based IDDM prevention trial. *Diabetes* 1997; **46**: 557–564.
10. Virtanen S, Jaakkola L, Räsänen L *et al.* Nitrate and nitrite intake and the risk for type 1 diabetes in Finnish children. *Diabetic Med* 1994; **11**: 656–662.
11. Kostraba JN, Cay EC, Rewers M *et al.* Nitrate levels in community drinking water and risk of IDDM. *Diabetes Care* 1992; **15**: 1505–1508.
12. Skyler JS, Marks JB. Immune intervention in Type 1 diabetes mellitus. *Diabetes Rev* 1993; **1**: 15–42.

13. Harrison L. IDDM prevention reaches new heights in Orvieto. *Diabetes Prev Ther* 1996; **10**(1): 1–2.
14. Åkerblom HK, Knip M, Simell O. From pathomechanisms to prediction, prevention and improved care of insulin-dependent diabetes mellitus in children. *Ann Med* 1997; **29**: 383–385.
15. Knip M. Disease-associated autoimmunity and prevention of insulin-dependent diabetes mellitus. *Ann Med* 1997; **29**: 447–451.
16. Notkins AL. Intervention for diabetes prevention at neonatal age. *Diabetes Metab Rev* 1998; **14**: 109–110.
17. Pozzilli P. Prevention of insulin-dependent diabetes mellitus 1998. *Diabetes Metab Rev* 1998; **14**: 69–84.
18. American Diabetes Association. Prevention of type 1 diabetes mellitus. *Diabetes Care* 1996; **19**: 545.
19. Elliot RB, Mandrup-Poulsen T. The Use of Nicotinamide to Prevent Type 1 Diabetes. In Palmer JP (ed.). *Prediction, Prevention and Genetic Counseling in IDDM*. Chichester: Wiley, 1996; 238–292.
20. Goodman LS, Gilman A. *The Pharmacological Basis of Therapeutics*. New York: Macmillan, 1975; 1554–1556.
21. Andersen HU, Jorgensen KH, Egeberg J, Mandrup-Poulsen T, Nerup J. Nicotinamide prevents interleukin-1 effects on insulin release and nitric production in rat islets of Langerhans. *Diabetes* 1994; **43**: 770–777.
22. Pan J, Chan EK, Cheta D, Schranz V, Charles MA. The effects of nicotinamide and glimepiride on diabetes prevention in BB rats. *Life Sci* 1995; **57**: 1525–1532.
23. Lazarus SS, Shapiro SH. Influence of nicotinamide and pyridine nucleotides on streptozotocin and alloxan induced pancreatic B cell toxicity. *Diabetes* 1973; **22**: 499–506.
24. Gorbenko N, Poltorack V, Gladkih A, Borodina D. Nicotinamide prevents the development of insulin deficiency in streptozotocin-treated newborn rats. *Diabetologia* 1997; **40** (Suppl 1): A68.
25. Yamada K, Nonaka K, Hanfusa T, Miyazaki A, Toyoshima H, Tarui S. Preventive and therapeutic effects of large-dose nicotinamide injections on diabetes associated with insulitis. *Diabetes* 1982; **31**: 749–753.
26. Elliot RB, Pilcher CC. Prevention of diabetes in normal school children. *Diabetes Res Clin Pract* 1991; **14**: 585.
27. Elliot RB, Pilcher CC, Stewart A, Fergusson D, McGregory MA. The use of nicotinamide in the prevention of Type 1 diabetes. Immunosuppressive and antiinflammatory drugs. *Ann NY Acad Sci* 1993; **696**: 333–341.
28. Elliot RB, Chase HP. Prevention or delay of type 1 (insulin dependent) diabetes mellitus in children using nicotinamide. *Diabetologia* 1991: **34**: 362–365.
29. Herskowitz RD, Jackson RA, Soeldner JS, Eisenbarth GS. Pilot trial to

prevent Type 1 diabetes: Progression to overt IDDM despite oral nicotinamide. *J Autoimmun* 1989; **2**: 733–737.

30. The IMDIAB Group. Multi-center randomised trial at different doses of nicotinamide in patients with recent-onset IDDM. *Diabetologia* 1997; **40** (Suppl 1): A68.

31. Pozzilli P on behalf of the IMDIAB Group. BCG vaccine in insulin-dependent diabetes mellitus. *Lancet* 1997; **349**: 1520–1521.

32. Moore WP, Gale EAM and the ENDIT Group. Feasibility of a multi-national diabetes prevention trial in first degree relatives of a child with IDDM. *Diabetologia* 1997; **40** (Suppl 1): A67.

33. Honeyman M, Wasserfall C, Nerup J, Rossini A. Prediction and prevention of IDDM. *Diabetologia* 1997; **40** (Suppl 3): B58–B61.

34. Elliot RB, Berryman CC, Crossley JR, James AG. Partial preservation of pancreatic beta-cell function in children with diabetes. *Lancet* 1981; **ii**: 1–4.

35. Mistura L, Beccaria L, Meschi F, D'Arcais A, Pellini C, Puzzovio M, Chiumello G. Prednisone treatment in newly diagnosed type 1 diabetic children: 1 year followup. *Diabetes Care* 1981; **10**: 39–43.

36. Mahon JL, Dupre J. Cyclosporine and Azathioprine for IDDM. In Palmer JP (ed.). *Prediction, Prevention and Genetic Counselling in IDDM*. Chichester: Wiley, 1996; 257–271.

37. Feutren G, Papoz L, Assan R *et al.* Cyclosporin increases the rate and length of remissions in insulin-dependent diabetes of recent onset. *Lancet* 1986; **ii**: 119–123.

38. The Canadian-European Randomized Control Trial Group. Cyclosporin-induced remission of IDDM after early intervention. *Diabetes* 1988; **37**: 1574–1582.

39. Skyler J, Rabinovitch A. Cyclosporin in recent onset type 1 diabetes mellitus. Effects on islet beta-cell function. *J Diabet Complications* 1992: **6**: 77–88.

40. Chase HP, Butler-Simon N, Garg SK *et al.* Cyclosporine A for treatment of new-onset insulin-dependent diabetes mellitus. *Paediatrics* 1990; **85**: 241–245.

41. Cook JJ, Hudson I, Harrison LC *et al.* A double-blind controlled trial of azathioprine in children with newly diagnosed type 1 diabetes. *Diabetes* 1989; **38**: 779–783.

42. Silverstein J, Maclaren N, Riley W, Spiller R, Radjenovic D, Johnson S. Immunosuppression with azathioprine and prednisone in recent-onset insulin-dependent diabetes mellitus. *N Engl J Med* 1983; **319**: 599–604.

43. Füchtenbush M, Ziegler AG. Prophylactic Insulin Treatment in Pre-Type-1-Diabetes. In Marshall SM, Home PD, Rizza RA (eds). *The Diabetes Annual/10*. Amsterdam: Elsevier, 1996; 135–147.

44. Ramiya VK, Maclaren NK. Insulin in diabetes prevention. *Horm Res* 1997; **48** (Suppl 4): 67–70.
45. Christie MR, Brown TJ, Cassidy D. Binding of antibodies in sera from Type 1 (insulin-dependent) diabetic patients to glutamate decarboxylase from rat tissues. Evidence for antigenic and non-antigenic forms of the enzyme. *Diabetologia* 1992; **35**: 380–384.
46. Rabin DU, Pleasic SM, Shapiro JA *et al*. Islet cell antigen 512 is a diabetes-specific islet autoantigen related to protein tyrosine phosphatases. *J Immunol* 1994; **152**: 3183–3188.
47. Ziegler AG, Ziegler R, Vardi P, Jackson RA, Soeldner JS, Eisenbarth GS. Life table analysis of progression to diabetes of anti-insulin autoantibody positive relatives of Type 1 diabetics. *Diabetes* 1989; **38**: 1320–1325.
48. Hummel M, Durinovic-Bello I, Standl C, Ziegler AG. Cellular immune response to islet cell antigens in Type 1 diabetes (IDDM). *Diabetes* 1995; **44** (Suppl 1): 79A.
49. Wegmann DR, Gill RG, Norbury-Glaser M, Schloot N, Daniel D. Analysis of the spontaneous T-cell response to insulin in NOD mice. *J Autoimmun* 1994; **7**: 833–834.
50. Coutant R, Carel JC, Timsit J, Boitard C, Bougneres P. Insulin and the prevention of insulin-dependent diabetes mellitus. *Diabete Metab* 1997; **23** (Suppl 3): 25–28.
51. Appel MC, O'Neil JJ. Prevention of spontaneous diabetes in the bb/w rat by insulin treatment. *Pancreas* 1986; **1**: 356.
52. Orban T, Jackson R. Insulin Treatment in Pre-diabetes. In Palmer JP (ed.). *Prediction, Prevention and Genetic Counseling in IDDM*. Chichester: Wiley, 1996; 273–282.
53. Gotfredsen CF, Buschard K, Frandsen EK. Reduction of diabetes incidence of BB Wistar rats by early prophylactic insulin treatment of diabetes-prone animals. *Diabetologia* 1985; **28**: 933–935.
54. Like AA. Insulin injections prevent diabetes (DB) in Bio-Breeding/Worchester (BB/Wor) rats. *Diabetes* 1986; **35** (Suppl 1): 74A.
55. Atkinson MA, Maclaren NK, Luchetta R. Insulitis and diabetes in NOD mice reduced by prophylactic insulin therapy. *Diabetes* 1990; **39**: 933–937.
56. Thivolet CH, Goillot JE, Bedossa P, Durand A, Bonnard M, Orgiazzi J. Insulin prevents adoptive cell transfer of diabetes in autoimmune non-obese diabetic mouse. *Diabetologia* 1991; **34**: 314–319.
57. Muir A, Peck A, Clare-Salzler M *et al*. Insulin immunization of NOD mice induces a protective insulitis characterised by diminished intra-islet interferon-γ transcription. *Diabetes* 1993; **42** (Suppl 1): 5A.
58. Karounos DG, Bryson JS, Cohen DA. Metabolically inactive insulin analog prevents type I diabetes in prediabetic NOD mice. *J Clin Invest* 1997; **100**: 1344–1348.

59. Karlsson FA, Bjork E. Beta-cell rest: a strategy for the prevention of autoimmune diabetes. *Autoimmunity* 1997; **26**: 117–122.

60. Keller RJ, Eisenbarth GS, Jackson RA. Insulin prophylaxis in individuals at high risk of type 1 diabetes. *Lancet* 1993; **341**: 927–928.

61. Rodríguez-Villar C, Conget I, Vidal J *et al*. A pilot trial of insulin administration in the prediabetic state. *Diabetologia* 1995; **38** (Suppl 1): A99.

62. Füchtenbusch M, Rabl W, Grassl B, Bachmann W, Standl E, Ziegler A-G. Delay of Type 1 diabetes in high risk, first degree relatives by parenteral antigen administration: the Schwabing Insulin Prophylaxis Pilot Trial. *Diabetologia* 1998; **41**: 536–541.

63. The DPT-1 Study Group. The Diabetes Prevention Trial—Type 1 Diabetes (DPT-1): Implementation of Screening and Staging of Relatives. *Diabetes* 1995; **44** (Suppl 1): 129A.

64. DPT-1 Study Group. The Diabetes Prevention Trial—Type 1 Diabetes (DPT-1): Enrollment Report. *Diabetes* 1997; **46** (Suppl 1): 163A.

65. DPT-1 Study Group. The Diabetes Prevention Trial—Type 1 Diabetes (DPT-1): Progress Report. *Diabetologia* 1997; **40** (Suppl 1): A66.

66. Weiner HL. Oral Tolerance. In Palmer JP (ed.). *Prediction, Prevention and Generic Counseling in IDDM*. Chichester: Wiley, 1996; 293–315.

67. Brandtzaeg P. Overview of the mucosal immune system. *Curr Tops Microbiol Immunol* 1983; **13**: 138–142.

68. Mattingly JA. Immunological suppression after oral administration of antigen. III Activation of suppressor-inducer cells in the Peyer's patches. *Cell Immunol* 1984; **86**: 46–52.

69. Husby S, Jensenius JC, Svehag S-E. Passage of undegraded dietary antigen into the blood of healthy adults. Further characterisation of the kinetics of uptake and the size distribution of the antigen. *Scand J Immunol* 1986; **24**: 447–452.

70. Weiner HL, Friedman A, Miller A *et al*. Oral tolerance: immunologic mechanisms and treatment of murine and human organ specific auto-immune diseases by oral administration of autoantigens. *Annu Rev Immunol* 1994; **12**: 809–837.

71. Miller A, Lider O, Weiner HL. Antigen-driven bystander suppression following oral administration of antigens. *J Exp Med* 1991; **174**: 791–798.

72. Karjalainen J, Martin JM, Knip M *et al*. A bovine albumin peptide as a possible trigger of insulin-dependent diabetes mellitus. *N Engl J Med* 1992; **327**: 302–307.

73. Zhang Z, Micheal JG. Orally inducible immune unresponsiveness is abrogated by INF-γ treatment. *J Immunol* 1990; **144**: 4163–4165.

74. Bland P. MHC class II expression by the gut epithelium. *Immunol Today* 1988; **9**: 174–178.

75. Higgins P, Weiner HL. Suppression of experimental autoimmune encephalomyelitis by oral administration of myelin basic protein and its fragments. *J Immunol* 1988; **140**: 440–445.
76. Nagler-Anderson C, Bober LA, Robinson ME, Siskind GW, Thorbecke FJ. Suppression of type II collagen induced arthritis by intragastric administration of soluble type II collagen. *Proc Natl Acad Sci USA*. 1986; **83**: 7443–7446.
77. Salen E. Experiments on the oral administration of insulin. *Acta Med Scand* 1924; **60**: 74.
78. Walton RP, Basset EF. Enteral absorption of insulin. *Proc Soc Exp Biol Med* 1933; **30**: 1184.
79. Shichiri M, Okada A, Karasaki K, Kawamori R, Shigeta Y, Abe H. Increase in plasma immunoreactive insulin following administration of insulin to the gastrointestinal tract of rabbits. *Diabetes* 1972; **21**: 203.
80. Shichiri M, Kawamori R, Yoshida M *et al.* Short-term treatment of alloxan-diabetic rats with intrajejunal administration of water-in-oil-in-water insulin-emulsions. *Diabetes* 1975; **24**: 971.
81. Kelly WA. Passage of insulin through the wall of the gastrointestinal tract of the infant mouse. *Nature* 1961; **186**: 971.
82. Pierce AE, Risdall PC, Shaw B. Absorption of orally administered insulin by the newly born calf. *J Physiol* 1964; **171**: 203.
83. Danforth E, Moore RO. Intestinal absorption of insulin in the rat. *Endocrinology* 1959; **65**: 118.
84. Crane CW, Luntz GRWN. Absorption of insulin from the human small intestine. *Diabetes* 1968; **17**: 625.
85. Zhang ZJ, Davidson L, Eisenbarth GS, Weiner HL. Suppression of diabetes in non-obese diabetic mice by oral administration of porcine insulin. *Proc Natl Acad Sci USA* 1991; **88**: 10252–10256.
86. Muir A, Schatz D, Maclaren N. Antigen-specific immunotherapy: oral tolerance and subcutaneous immunization in the treatment of insulin-dependent-diabetes. *Diabetes Metab Rev* 1993; **9**: 279–287.
87. Bergerot I, Fabien N, Maguer V, Thivolet C. Oral administration of human insulin to NOD mice generates CD4+ T cells that suppress adoptive transfer of diabetes. *J Autoimmun* 1994; **7**: 655–663.
88. Hancock WW, Polanski M, Zhang J, Blogg N, Weiner HL. Suppression of insulitis in Non-Obese Diabetic (NOD) mice by oral insulin administration is associated with selective expression of Interleukin-4 and -10, transforming growth factor-β, and prostaglandin-E. *Am J Pathol* 1995; **147**: 1193–1199.
89. Ploix C, Bergerot I, Fabien N, Perschi S, Moulin V, Thivolet C. Protection against autoimmune diabetes with oral insulin is associated with the

presence of IL-4 type 2 T-cells in the pancreas and pancreatic lymph nodes. *Diabetes* 1998; **47**: 39–44.

90. Hartmann B, Bellmann K, Ghiea I, Kleemann R, Kolb H. Oral insulin for diabetes prevention in NOD mice: potentiation by enhancing Th2 cytokine expression in the gut through bacterial adjuvant. *Diabetologia* 1997; **40**: 902–909.

91. Bergerot I, Moulin V, Fabien N, Ploix C, Czerkinsky C, Thivolet C. CTB-insulin conjugates potentiate oral tolerance against autoimmune diabetes in NOD mice. *Diabetes* 1996; **45** (Suppl 2): 83A.

92. Sobel DO, Yankelevich B, Goyal D, Nelson D, Mazumder A. The B-subunit of cholera toxin induces immunoregulatory cells and prevents diabetes in the NOD mouse. *Diabetes* 1998; **47**: 186–191.

93. Mordes JP, Schirf B, Roipko D *et al.* Oral insulin does not prevent insulin-dependent diabetes mellitus in BB rats. *Ann NY Acad Sci* 1996; **778**: 418–421.

94. Bellmann K, Kolb H, Rastegar S, Jee P, Scott FW. Potential risk of oral insulin with adjuvant for the prevention of Type I diabetes: a protocol effective in NOD mice may exacerbate disease in BB rats. *Diabetologia* 1998; **41**: 844–847.

95. Schatz D for the DPT-1 Study Group. The Diabetes Prevention Trial—Type 1 Diabetes (DPT-1): design and implementation of the oral antigen (insulin) protocol. *Diabetes* 1995; **44** (Suppl 1): 230A.

96. Falorni A, Örtquist E, Persson B, Lernmark Å. Radioimmunoassays for glutamic acid decarboxylase (GAD 65) and GAD 65 autoantibodies using 35S or 3H recombinant human ligands. *J Immunol Methods* 1995; **186**: 89–99.

97. Vardi P, Dib SA, Tuttleman M *et al.* Competitive insulin autoantibody assay. Prospective evaluation of subjects at high risk for development of type I diabetes mellitus. *Diabetes* 1987; **36**: 1286–1291.

98. Schmidli RS, Colman PG, Bonifacio E and participating laboratories. Disease sensitivity and specificity of 52 assays for glutamic acid decarboxylase antibodies: The Second International GAD Ab Workshop. *Diabetes* 1995; **44**: 636–640.

99. Bingley PJ, Colman PG, Eisenbarth GS *et al.* Standardisation of IVGTT to predict IDDM. *Diabetes Care* 1992; **15**: 1313–1316.

100. Jertborn M, Svennerholm AM, Holmgren J. Safety and immunogenicity of an oral recombinant cholera B subunit-whole cell vaccine in Swedish volunteers. *Vaccine* 1992; **10**: 130.

101. Begue RE, Castellares G, Ruiz R *et al.* Community-based assessment of safety and immunogenicity of the whole cell plus recombinant B subunit (WC/rBS) oral cholera vaccine in Peru. *Vaccine* 1995; **13**: 691.

102. Skyler JS, Marks JB. Future Approaches to Prevention. In Palmer JR (ed.). *Prediction, Prevention and Genetic Counseling in IDDM*. Chichester: Wiley, 1996; 369–389.

103. Harrison LC, Dempsey-Collier M, Takahashi K, Angstein P, Kramer DR. Prevention of insulin-dependent diabetes by CD8$\gamma\delta$T cells induced by aerosol insulin. *Diabetologia* 1997; **40** (Suppl 1): A67.

5

Overview of the Etiopathogenesis of Type 2 Diabetes Mellitus

The ominous increase in the incidence of type 2 diabetes mellitus in the contemporary world, especially in developing countries, was mentioned in the Introduction. There is a lot of data related to its causes and mechanisms but these are still insufficient. Type 2 diabetes can be considered a multifactorial and heterogeneous disorder[1-3].

As in Chapter 2, this chapter will present the principal aspects of the etiopathogenesis of type 2 diabetes that will help in the discussions of the problems of prophylaxis as clearly and succinctly as possible.

5.1   GENETIC BACKGROUND

The important role of genetics in the production of diabetes mellitus has been demonstrated by numerous arguments[4]. It is known for example, that type 2 diabetes has a strong family basis and it has been estimated that almost 40% of the siblings of patients can expect to develop the disease, assuming a maximum life expectancy of 80 years[5,6]. Some twin studies indicate that there is about 90% concordance for type 2 diabetes[7]. Population-based studies of the peculiarities of the genetics of type 2 diabetes in some ethnic groups have been very interesting. A good example is the observation that a high efficiency in the metabolism of carbohydrates has been an evolutionary advantage in peoples that have traditionally lived with difficult nutritional conditions; once these populations adopt a sedentary lifestyle and a diet with an excess of calories, sugar and saturated fats they seem to be more predisposed to disorders of glucose metabolism (the "thrifty gene" hypothesis)[6,8,9]. Animal models of type 2 diabetes (the ob/ob and db/db mice and other models) and specific genetic syndromes that include glucose intolerance provide additional information on the role of genetics in type 2 diabetes[1,4]. Recent advances in molecular genetics have enabled the recognition of the genes involved in some subtypes of type 2 diabetes with a well defined mode of inheritance and a strong association with genetic factors[10].

However, the number of genes involved in NIDDM and their mode of inheritance are still unclear. At present, over 250 candidate genes have been studied for linkage or association to type 2 diabetes[2]. Amongst these are the insulin gene (and its 5' flanking region); the insulin receptor gene; the glucokinase gene; genes coding for Glut 1, Glut 2 and Glut 4; the HLA region; the glycogen synthase gene and a number of genes involved in lipid metabolism[3]. Unfortunately, none of these linkages or associations have been shown to be significant within a given ethnic group or to differ across ethnic lines[6].

Other investigators have undertaken genome-wide searches to identify potential susceptibility loci for type 2 diabetes[2,4,6,11]. Thus, evidence for linkage to markers on chromosome 2 have been found (in Mexican Americans), on chromosomes 6 and 11 (in Mexican Americans), on chromosomes 1, 4 and 7 (in Pima Indians), on chromosome 7 (in Europids), on chromosome 12 (in Finns)[6,11]. Recent advances in positional cloning have raised hopes for the eventual identification of the gene or genes responsible for human type 2 diabetes[12].

The location of such a gene or genes will be a major step towards the precise identification of individuals at risk for type 2 diabetes and targeting of intense preventive measures. At the moment, the most important element for prevention is the modification of the environmental factors associated with the risk of type 2 diabetes[6].

5.2   ENVIRONMENTAL FACTORS

The list of diabetogenic agents is growing rapidly. Obesity and lack of physical activity, age, stress and the so-called "modern lifestyle" remain some of the most significant factors[1,2]. Paul Zimmet's highly suggestive statements are worthy of mention. He talked recently of "Coca Cola-nization" of some communities and called diabetes "a Western killer let loose in Paradise" (cited in reference 3).

5.2.1   Obesity and Nutritional Errors

The diabetogenic role of obesity has been known for a long time and has been confirmed by numerous cross-sectional and longitudinal studies. Approximately 75–80% of patients with type 2 diabetes have been or are obese. High BMI seems to be associated with increased risk of diabetes in both sexes and all ethnic groups[6]. Both the total fat content of the body and its distribution are important[2]. Intra-abdominal fat accumulation (central or abdominal obesity) acts as an independent diabetogenic factor, as can be confirmed by the results of studies from the USA, Mauritius, Finland and Sweden[6]. It is possible that the overall body mass predominantly influences insulin secretion while abdominal obesity is more closely related to insulin resistance[13]. The deleterious effect of intra-abdominal fat tissue has been attributed to its high lipolytic rate, which results in elevated portal and peripheral levels of free fatty acids leading to hepatic and muscle resistance respectively[14].

A Western-style, high-fat, low-carbohydrate, low-fiber diet predisposes to obesity and is associated with type 2 diabetes. The nutritional risk factors responsible for this interact with each other in a complex way. Dietary sugar does not on its own produce obesity or type 2 diabetes but in large quantities can aggravate hyperglycemia in decompensated diabetes[15].

5.2.2   Physical Activity

Reduced physical activity is another factor that has been associated with insulin resistance and type 2 diabetes[1,2,15]; conversely, physical training has been shown to improve insulin action. A close correlation between the maximum aerobic power ($VO_{2(max)}$) and whole body insulin-mediated glucose disposal has been noted in both non-diabetic and diabetic individuals[2,16]. It is noteworthy that type 2 diabetes patients have a consistently lower $VO_{2(max)}$ than non-diabetic subjects of similar age and body weight and part of the insulin resistance in type 2 diabetes is the result of decreased physical training[2].

5.2.3   Age

It is well established that the prevalence of impaired glucose tolerance (IGT) and type 2 diabetes increase with advancing age[17]. The glucose intolerance of aging is demonstrated primarily by an increase in the postprandial blood glucose and insulin response to an oral glucose challenge as well as to a mixed meal[18]. Fasting blood glucose levels are generally not significantly elevated. The increase in postprandial blood glucose concentrations may be more important in women than in men.

This kind of glucose intolerance appears to be due to an increase in peripheral insulin resistance that occurs with aging. The precise mechanisms of this disorder remain unknown, but are probably associated with post-receptor defect(s) in insulin action. Subtle abnormalities of insulin release, insulin binding and hepatic glucose suppression by insulin may exist but they do not appear to play a major role in glucose intolerance of age. Changes in the degree of physical activity and increases in abdominal adiposity may underlie part of the insulin resistance noted in elderly people. The loss of lean body mass is not as relevant[17].

5.2.4   Other Factors

Commencing from the "thrifty genotype" hypothesis mentioned above, it has been suggested that a "thrifty phenotype" hypothesis offers a more satisfactory explanation of the epidemiology of type 2 diabetes[19]. The essence of this is that poor nutrition in fetal and early infant life is detrimental to the mechanisms maintaining carbohydrate tolerance. It is suggested that the undernourished fetus makes metabolic adjustments which benefit it in the short term by increasing fuel availability but that these adaptations become permanently programmed, persisting throughout life and determining insulin resistance. Thus, insulin resistance may be considered as a price of short-term successful adaptation to under-nutrition *in utero*. Under-nutrition may also affect the structure and function of the islet beta cells. Although these early changes determine susceptibility, additional factors such as obesity, physical inactivity and aging further increase insulin resistance and play a role in the time of onset and severity of type 2 diabetes. The "thrifty phenotype" hypothesis also explains the clustering of other disorders such as hypertension with diabetes in the X syndrome. These different abnormalities are related because they have a common origin in suboptimal development of particular stages of intrauterine life[20]. The studies confirming a linkage between poor early growth and loss of glucose tolerance or the presence of the insulin resistance syndrome were carried out on different population groups (including Pima Indians in the USA, Swedish men, Danish twins, Australian Aborigines)[21].

Smoking has been shown to be associated with the development of insulin resistance, which can be reversed by the cessation of smoking[22]. The mechanisms responsible for the influence of smoking on insulin sensitivity have yet to be clarified[3]. Alterations in sympathetic nervous system activity have been suggested as the cause of the insulin resistance, but one also could argue that reduced physical activity due to the adverse effects of smoking on the respiratory and cardiovascular systems is responsible[2].

The contributions and mechanisms of action of psychosocial stress are being investigated with increasing attention[23].

A possible connection between breastfeeding practices and the risk of type 2 diabetes has also been mentioned[24].

Most of the factors discussed above can be classified under the heading of "modern lifestyle". Recognizing the role of the modern lifestyle in diabetes gives us a promising prophylactic perspective.

5.3 PATHOGENESIS

Although the pathogenesis of type 2 diabetes mellitus has many controversial aspects, it is thought that two major defects—insulin resistance and impaired beta-cell function—must be present simultaneously. Whichever defect initiates the disease, it will lead to the emergence of the other abnormality. Both of these defects can have a genetic as well as an acquired component[2].

5.3.1 Impaired Insulin Secretion

In the early stages of type 2 diabetes, the absolute basal insulin levels are normal or even elevated, but are inappropriately low in comparison with the raised blood glucose concentrations[15]. Recent investigations have shown that much of the "insulin" measured by conventional assays is in fact composed of the abnormal cleavage products of proinsulin. Most type 2 diabetes patients probably have an absolute insulin deficiency. The pulsatility of basal insulin secretion is abnormal in type 2 diabetes, possibly rendering the insulin less biologically effective[2,15].

The first phase of insulin secretion in response to glucose is deficient in type 2 diabetes, producing postprandial hyperglycemia through insulin deficiency and lack of the priming effects of the first-phase insulin in the target organs[25]. The response to non-glucose stimuli is normal, suggesting a specific glucose receptor derangement[15].

With persistent hyperglycemia the second phase of insulin release in response to glucose becomes attenuated in type 2 diabetes.

The relationship between the plasma glucose concentration and the insulin response is complex and resembles an inverted U or a horse shoe. As this curve resembles Starling's curve of the heart, DeFronzo referred to it as "Starling's curve of the pancreas"[2,26]. In normal-weight subjects with impaired glucose tolerance and mild diabetes mellitus, plasma insulin response to ingested glucose increases progressively until the fasting glucose values reach about 6.7 mmol/l. Thereafter, further increases in fasting glucose concentrations are associated with a progressive decline in insulin secretion, which could indicate a toxic effect of glucose on beta-cell function. The same curve depicts the relationship between fasting plasma insulin and glucose concentration[15].

With the onset of insulinopenia, whether relative or absolute, marked fasting hyperglycemia will ensue due to excessive glucose production by the liver and a further decrease in tissue glucose clearance. Another important pathogenetic disturbance which appears at the same time as the onset of insulinopenia is a post-receptor defect in insulin action. The final clinical picture would be that of typical type 2 diabetes[2].

5.3.2 Insulin Resistance

This is a nearly universal phenomenon in patients with established type 2 diabetes[1,2,15,16]. However, many prospective studies have clearly shown that hyperinsulinemia and insulin resistance precede the development of IGT and that IGT is the forerunner of type 2 diabetes[2,27,28]. Such results provide conclusive evidence that insulin resistance is the inherited defect that initiates the diabetic state in most type 2 diabetics[2].

The basic condition responsible for insulin resistance remains unclear. Attention has been concentrated on some intracellular disturbances involving glucose metabolism—such as insulin receptor signal transduction, glucose transport, glucose phosphorylation, glycogen synthase activity. There are also other possible explanations, such as abnormalities in intracellular lipid metabolism, enhanced sympathetic nervous system activity, disturbances in muscle blood flow on fiber type, alterations in ion pump activity. As has been underlined by DeFronzo and his co-workers, all these abnormalities could represent the primary or inherited (genetic) defect in type 2 diabetes[2].

Regardless of the cause(s) of the insulin resistance, the beta cell will increase its secretion of insulin to offset the defect in insulin action. The resultant compensatory hyperinsulinemia will downregulate different intracellular events involved in insulin action and thus serve as a self-perpetuating factor of insulin resistance. Eventually, beta-cell exhaustion will result.

5.3.3 Combined Defects

In principle, it is possible that the disorders in insulin action (involving both muscle and the liver) and insulin secretion result from the same, unidentified, genetic abnormality and that insulin resistance and impaired beta-cell activity develop in parallel[2].

5.4 THE HISTOLOGY OF THE PANCREAS IN TYPE 2 DIABETES

Total islet mass and beta-cell number are reduced to 50–60% of normal in type 2 diabetes[15]. However, an increase in mass of the glucagon-producing α cells may be observed (Table 5.1).

The most important histologic aspect is amyloid deposition in the islets. Amyloidosis is not specific to diabetes; however, it is far more common and severe in type 2 diabetes than in non-diabetics. Islet amyloid occurs only in islets containing insulin-producing cells[29]. It was found that the major constituent of the amyloid fibrils is a peptide, designated islet amyloid polypeptide or amylin[30]. This has 50% homology with the regulatory peptide, calcitonin-gene-related peptide and there is evidence that it originates in the beta-cell secretory granules[15,29].

5.5 PRINCIPLES OF PROPHYLAXIS

Table 5.2 lists the principal causes and mechanisms involved in the production of type 2 diabetes mellitus based on the strategies and projects for prevention of this disease that can be designed.

If we commence from the observation that type 2 diabetes is a multifactorial and heterogeneous disorder, for prophylaxis to be truly

Table 5.1. Pancreatic morphologic features in type 2 diabetes

Macroscopy
  Without significant anomalies
Microscopy
  Reduction in total islet mass
  Reduction in beta-cell mass
  Increase in the mass of the glucagon-producing α cells
  Islet amyloidosis (islet hyalinization)
  Islet fibrosis
  Beta-cell degranulation
  Hydropic degeneration

Adapted from references 15 and 29

Table 5.2. Causes of and mechanisms involved in the production of type 2 diabetes mellitus

Genetic component
Environmental factors:
Obesity
Reduced physical activity
Age
Stress
Smoking
Other factors
Insulin resistance
Abnormal insulin secretion
Combined defects

efficient it must be based on the simultaneous modification of several potential risk factors. Nevertheless, existing data suggests that even one intervention (for example weight loss or increased physical activity) can lead to a decrease in the incidence of type 2 diabetes[6].

In the present situation, two components of primary prevention could be considered:

1. A population-based approach to lifestyle change and the modification of those environmental agents that are the underlying causes of type 2 diabetes.
2. A high-risk approach for screening subjects at especially increased risk of developing the disease and bringing preventive care to them[5,31].

In fact, the population and high-risk strategies are generally complementary[31,32]. Although the population approach may be more useful in countries with increased genetic susceptibility (in which case the two strategies are effectively the same), the high-risk alternative may present advantages in communities of low or moderate genetic risk, as well as in communities in which type 2 diabetes is not the predominant non-communicable disease. The high-risk strategy must also be entertained while there is still uncertainty as to whether the relationship between risk factors and disease is really causal[6].

The results obtained till now and the problems raised by the prevention of type 2 diabetes mellitus will be the object of discussion of Chapter 6.

REFERENCES

1. Weir GC, Leahy JL. Pathogenesis of Non-Insulin-Dependent (Type II) Diabetes Mellitus. In Kahn CR, Weir GS (eds). *Joslin's Diabetes Mellitus*, 13th edn. Philadelphia: Lea & Febiger, 1994; 240–264.
2. DeFronzo RA, Bonadonna RC, Ferrannini E. Pathogenesis of NIDDM. In Alberti KGMM, Zimmet P, DeFronzo RA, Keen H (eds). *International Textbook of Diabetes Mellitus*, 2nd edn. Chichester: Wiley, 1997; 635–711.
3. Bloomgarden ZT. International Diabetes Federation Meeting 1997. Type 2 diabetes: its prevalence, causes and treatment. *Diabetes Care* 1998; **21**: 860–865.
4. Scheuner MT, Raffel LJ, Rotter JI. Genetics of Diabetes. In Alberti KGMM, Zimmet P, DeFronzo RA, Keen H (eds). *International Textbook of Diabetes Mellitus*, 2nd edn. Chichester: Wiley, 1997; 37–88.
5. Köbberling J, Tilil H. Empirical Risk Figures for First-degree Relatives of Non-insulin-dependent Diabetes. In Köbberling J, Tattersal R (eds). *The Genetics of Diabetes Mellitus*. London: Academic Press, 1982; 201–210.
6. Tuomilheto J, Tuomilehto-Wolf E, Zimmet P, Alberti KGMM, Knowler WC. Primary Prevention of Diabetes Mellitus. In Alberti KGMM, Zimmet P, DeFronzo RA, Keen H (eds). *International Textbook of Diabetes Mellitus*, 2nd edn. Chichester: Wiley, 1997; 1799–1827.
7. Barnett AH, Eff C, Leslie RDG, Pyke DA. Diabetes in identical twins: a study of 200 pairs. *Diabetologia* 1981; **20**: 87–93.
8. Neel JV. Diabetes mellitus: a "thrifty" genotype rendered detrimental by "progress"? *Am J Hum Genet* 1962; **14**: 353–362.
9. Zimmet P, Serjeantson S, Dowse G, Finch C, Collins V. Diabetes Mellitus and Cardiovascular Disease in Developing Populations—Hunter-Gatherers in the Fast Lane. In Gracey M, Kretchner N, Rossi A (eds). *Sugars in Nutrition*. Nestlé Nutrition Workshop Series, vol. 25. New York: Nestec, Vevey/Raven Press, 1991; 197–209.
10. Velho G, Froguel P. Genetic determinants of non-insulin-dependent diabetes mellitus: strategies and recent results. *Diabete Metab* 1997; **23**: 7–17.
11. Hanis CL, Boerwinkle E, Chakraborty R *et al.* A genome-wide search for human non-insulin-dependent (type 2) diabetes genes reveals a major susceptibility locus on chromosome 2. *Nat Genet* 1996; **13**: 161–166.

12. Collins FS. Positional cloning moves from perditional to traditional. *Nat Genet* 1995; **9**: 347–350.
13. Björntorp P. Abdominal obesity and the development of non-insulin-dependent diabetes mellitus. *Diabetes Metab Rev* 1988; **4**: 615–622.
14. Lonnquist F, Thorne A, Nilsell K, Hoffstedt J, Amer P. A pathogenetic role of visceral beta-adrenoreceptors in obesity. *J Clin Invest* 1995; **95**: 1109–1116.
15. Williams G, Pickup JC. *Handbook of Diabetes*. Oxford: Blackwell Science, 1998; **12**: 16.
16. Schneider SH, Morgado A. Effects of fitness and physical training on carbohydrate metabolism and associated cardiovascular risk factors in patients with diabetes. *Diabetes Rev* 1995; **3**: 379–403.
17. Peters AL, Davidson MB. Aging and Diabetes. In Alberti KGMM, Zimmet P, DeFronzo RA, Keen H (eds). *International Textbook of Diabetes Mellitus*, 2nd edn. Chichester: Wiley, 1997; 1151–1176.
18. Fraze E, Chiou M, Chen M, Chen I, Reaven GM. Age-related changes in postprandial plasma glucose, insulin and free fatty acid concentrations in non-diabetic individuals. *J Am Geriatr Soc* 1987; **35**: 224–228.
19. Hales CN, Barker DJP. Type 2 (non-insulin dependent) diabetes mellitus: the thrifty phenotype hypothesis. *Diabetologia* 1992; **35**: 595–601.
20. Phillips DIW, Hales CH. The Intrauterine Environment and Susceptibility to Non-insulin Dependent Diabetes and the Insulin Resistance Syndrome. In Marshall SM, Home PD, Rizza RA (eds). *The Diabetes Annual/10*. Amsterdam: Elsevier, 1996; 1–13.
21. Hales CN. Early growth retardation predisposes to maturity onset diabetes. *IDF Bull* 1998; **43**(2): 8–14.
22. Faccini FS, Hollenbeck CB, Jeppesen J, Chen YD, Reaven GM. Insulin resistance and cigarette smoking. *Lancet* 1992; **339**: 1128–1130.
23. Räikkönen K, Keltikangas-Järvinen L, Adlerereutz H, Hautanen A. Psychosocial stress and the insulin resistance syndrome. *Metabolism* 1996; **4**: 1533–1538.
24. Pettitt DJ, Forman MR, Hanson RL, Knowler WC, Bennett PH. Breast-feeding and incidence of non-insulin-dependent diabetes mellitus in Pima Indians. *Lancet* 1997; **350**: 166–168.
25. Bruce DG, Chisholm DJ, Storlien LH, Kraegen EW. Physiological importance of deficiency in early prandial insulin secretion in non-insulin dependent diabetes. *Diabetes* 1988; **37**: 736–744.
26. DeFronzo RA. Pathogenesis of type 2 (non-insulin dependent) diabetes mellitus: a balanced overview. *Diabetologia* 1992; **35**: 389–397.
27. DeFronzo RA. Lilly Lecture. The triumvirate: beta cell, muscle, liver. A collusion responsible for NIDDM. *Diabetes* 1988; **37**: 667–687.
28. Martin BC, Warram JH, Krolawski AS, Bergman RN, Soeldner JS, Kahn

RC. Role of glucose and insulin resistance in development of type 2 diabetes mellitus: results of a 25-year follow-up study. *Lancet* 1992; **340**: 925–929.

29. Klöppel G, In't Veld PA. Morphology of the Pancreas in Normal and Diabetic States. In Alberti KGMM, Zimmet P, DeFronzo RA, Keen H (eds). *International Textbook of Diabetes Mellitus*, 2nd edn. Chichester: Wiley, 1997; 287–313.

30. Johnson KH, O'Brien TD, Betsholtz C, Westermark P. Islet amyloid, islet-amyloid polypeptide, and diabetes mellitus. *N Engl J Med* 1989; **321**: 513–518.

31. *WHO Prevention of Diabetes Mellitus. Report of a WHO Study Group.* Geneva: World Health Organization, 1994.

32. Tuomilehto J, Wolf E. Primary prevention of diabetes mellitus. *Diabetes Care* 1987; **10**: 238–248.

6

Possibilities for Preventing Type 2 Diabetes Mellitus

6.1 INTRODUCTION

At first sight, the primary prophylaxis of type 2 diabetes mellitus appears simple: secondary and tertiary prophylaxis would seem to be more difficult. In reality, primary prevention raises many and difficult problems all over the world, bringing about—quite often—the failure of some promising projects. The clearest proof is the rapid increase in the number of cases in most countries.

The specialist literature of the last few years covers numerous works of a theoretical character intended to offer the most consistent support possible for practical antidiabetic activity and for prevention of the disease. Some data of a general nature will be presented in this first section.

An important premise for the prophylaxis of diabetes (not only of type 2) is the clear definition of its principal stages[1,2]. Thus, one may consider that the underlying process is genetic susceptibility. The first recognized stage (by current methods) is impaired glucose tolerance (IGT). This is followed by uncomplicated diabetes, where there is chronic hyperglycemia, and symptoms that may be attributable to hyperglycemia may or may not be present. From this stage, there may be a passage to diabetes with vascular complications, but without the associated manifestations or disability. The fourth stage is that of diabetes with disability, in which complications of diabetes determine functional impairment (Table 6.1). It must be underlined that progression through all these stages is not inevitable: in principle, intervention at any one stage may prevent progression to a later stage[2].

The knowledge about the genetic component of human type 2 diabetes has increased considerably (see Chapter 5) but therapeutic or preventive actions against the genetic determinants of this disease have not yet been taken into consideration. Nevertheless, some commentaries about this problem could be of practical use. Tuomilehto *et al.* emphasized that it is not type 2 diabetes but the *susceptibility* to type 2 diabetes that is inherited[3]. In individuals who have inherited predisposing genes, exposure to environmental risk factors can trigger the disease. This concept is based on the following arguments:

- Glucose tolerance (assessed by 2-hour post-challenge blood glucose) may deteriorate with age. This fact is negligible in subjects without genetic susceptibility to diabetes.
- In individuals with genetic susceptibility to diabetes, the slope of worsening of glucose tolerance varies. Usually, a flat line is seen in subjects who do not possess additional risk factors.
- The variation of slope in genetically predisposed individuals is determined by environmental and other genetic factors that often lead to insulin resistance.
- The influence of environmental risk factors may begin at any age. Their effect is likely to be associated with the duration and the amount of exposure[2].

The findings that different agents can induce significant levels of diabetes in subsequent generations and that the offspring of rats rendered diabetic with low-dose streptozotocin are insulin resistant

Table 6.1. A practical staging of diabetes mellitus

Genetic susceptibility
Impaired glucose tolerance (IGT)
Diabetes without complications
Diabetes with vascular complications
Diabetes with disability

Adapted from references 1 and 2

and can develop diabetes suggest that there may be complex interactions between susceptibility genes and the environmental factors of diabetes. Such interactions make work in this field more difficult than might at first be apparent[4–6].

Although prevention of type 1 diabetes is developing along the high-risk approach aimed at identifying and protecting susceptible individuals and a similar approach has been suggested for type 2 diabetes, it may well be that the population approach (which aims at identifying and controlling environmental factors of high incidence) will be more effective for type 2 diabetes[6–8]. As has been emphasized, these approaches should not conflict but the priority with a common disorder should be to discover and control the causes of incidence[8].

A critical evaluation of the evidence shows that 60–90% of the prevalence of diabetes is environmentally determined, an appraisal that has not been challenged[6,9]. Determination of the relative contribution made by the various factors under debate could provide direction for health education and health promotion. This could be useful in communities with high prevalence of diabetes in the same way as dietary improvement, physical exercise and avoidance of smoking contribute to the decrease of heart disease or lung cancer[6,10]. Boucher presented some of the available evidence for environmental causation or "triggering" of type 2 diabetes[6]. These are, briefly, that:

- It should be possible to produce type 2 diabetes in laboratory animals by exposure to certain environmental factors.
- There should be important geographic differences in the incidence of type 2 diabetes.
- In some populations, there should be rapid temporal changes in incidence in less than a generation which could not be accounted for by genetic change.
- The risk to immigrants of developing type 2 diabetes should rapidly rise to that of the host country.
- There should be strong epidemiological evidence that certain environmental factors induce type 2 diabetes in humans. Affluence, obesity and lack of exercise are associated with increased prevalence of human diabetes, and the role of increased exercise and weight loss in reducing the risk of diabetes has already been demonstrated[6,7,11].

As the World Health Organization has noted, intervention strategies for preventing type 2 diabetes are based on efforts to decrease insulin resistance and to promote and sustain islet beta-cell function (e.g. by programs of obesity reduction and the promotion of physical activity)[12]. It is felt that these measures are probably most usefully applied to high-risk subjects, amongst whom are:

- People with a strong family history of type 2 diabetes, including that with onset during youth.
- Those changing from traditional to Westernized lifestyles, from rural to urban societies or from active to sedentary lifestyles.
- People with a history of gestational diabetes mellitus, gestational impaired glucose tolerance or large-birth-weight babies.
- Those with other elements of the chronic metabolic syndrome (e.g. arterial hypertension, hyperlipoproteinemia and obesity—particularly central obesity).

The main lifestyle changes that reduce insulin resistance are:

- Correction and prevention of obesity.
- Avoidance of a high-fat diet (which leads to a decrease in energy consumption and increased insulin sensitivity).
- Derivation of a high proportion of the carbohydrate content of the diet from unrefined sources—soluble fiber should be included.
- Avoidance of, or cautious use of, diabetogenic drugs.
- Increased physical activity, which has a major beneficial effect on insulin sensitivity independent of its effect on weight.

In addition to targeting subjects at high risk, public education regarding lifestyle modification should be promoted on a wider scale, particularly in societies and communities with a high risk of developing type 2 diabetes.

The WHO also recommends that no prevention should be commenced without a properly constituted evaluation component. The principles and methods of evaluation are clearly presented in the WHO report of 1994[12].

Recent studies show that primary prevention of type 2 diabetes is possible. However, strategies for controlling the type 2 diabetes pandemic are still being developed[13–18]. Successful interventions to date have mainly relied upon control of obesity and increasing physical activity, although pharmacological agents are being studied.

Table 6.2. Essential directions in prevention of type 2 diabetes mellitus

---

Special position of IGT in type 2 diabetes prevention
Combating obesity and nutritional errors
Promotion of physical activity
Improving lifestyle
Combating other diabetogenic factors
New approaches to the problem
Particular aspects

While a mixture of both high-risk and population-based approaches is likely to be required, the former will not prevent new high-risk cases from developing. Unfortunately, the success in the primary prevention of cardiovascular disease through risk factor reduction has not controlled obesity, the most important risk factor for type 2 diabetes. New strategies are currently being implemented and focus upon modifications in the food supply of whole populations and a community development approach to altering attitudes to nutrition and exercise. These interventions are in the early stages of their development. For this reason, formative, process and quantitative evaluation remain essential components of any community-based program aimed at the primary prevention of type 2 diabetes[13]. The main points are listed in Table 6.2.

6.2 SPECIAL POSITION OF IGT IN TYPE 2 DIABETES PREVENTION

Impaired glucose tolerance is a major problem, not only as a result of its recognition as a first stage in the course of diabetes but also from the quantitative point of view[2]. Its prevalence increases with age: in the USA, for example, it reaches 23% of the population aged between 65 and 74 years[19]. It is a fact that the diagnosis, on a large scale, of these derangements utilizing WHO criteria presents real practical difficulties. In a synthesis of a large number of studies of diabetes in subjects with IGT, Tuomilehto *et al.* arrived at the conclusion that IGT does not indicate a discrete, stable condition or disease; however, IGT based on a single OGTT (without replication) clearly indicates a high risk for developing diabetes[2]. An analysis of six prospective population studies showed that BMI and fasting and post-load glucose concentrations measured at the time of IGT recognition were the most consistent and strongest predictors of progression from IGT to type 2 diabetes. This analysis indicates that people with IGT are at high risk of developing type 2 diabetes and that further assessment of risk can be made by other simple measurements. The ability to identify people at high risk of type 2 diabetes should facilitate clinical trials in diabetes prevention[20].

The initial efforts at preventive intervention in IGT have included a hypocaloric diet (for the obese subjects with IGT), exercise, sulfonylureas, biguanides, acarbose and troglitazone[2,21].

Two British studies established no discernible effect of either diet or oral hypoglycemic drugs on the incidence of subsequent diabetes, which did not differ significantly between treatment groups[22,23]. In another study, carried out in Sweden, individuals with IGT were randomly assigned to one of three groups, all of which received dietary therapy. The subjects in two of these groups also received either tolbutamide or placebo. Ten years later, the incidence of diabetes was lower in those treated with tolbutamide although the differences between the treatment groups were not statistically significant[24].

The 6-year Malmö feasibility study is related to the prevention of type 2 diabetes by diet and physical exercise[25]. From a previous 5-year screening program of 6956 47–49-year-old Malmö men, 41 with early-stage type 2 diabetes and 181 with IGT were selected for prospective study and to test the feasibility aspect of long-term intervention with an emphasis on lifestyle changes. A 5-year protocol, including an initial 6-month (randomized) pilot study, consisting of dietary treatment and/or increase in physical activity or training with annual check-ups, was completed by 90% of the subjects. Body weight was reduced by 2.3–3.7% among participants, whereas values increased by 0.5–1.7% in non-intervention subjects with IGT and in normal controls; maximal oxygen uptake was increased by 10–14% and decreased by 5–9% respectively. Glucose tolerance was normalized in >50% of subjects with IGT, the accumulated incidence of diabetes was 10.6% and more than 50% of the diabetics were in remission after a mean follow up of 6 years. Blood pressure, lipids and hyperinsulinemia were reduced and early insulin responsiveness to a glucose load was preserved. Improvement of glucose tolerance was correlated with weight reduction and increased fitness. Treatment was safe and mortality was low (in fact, 33% lower than in the remainder of the cohort). This study demonstrated the possibility of inducing and maintaining changes in lifestyle in a large group of IGT and type 2 diabetic subjects in the form of enduring weight loss, increased long-term physical activity and normalized age-related oxygen uptake. This would seem to prevent or postpone progression to diabetes in IGT subjects and delay metabolic deterioration in diabetic patients. The greatest benefit of intervention may not be improved glucose tolerance *per se*, but overall improvement in cardiovascular risk profile. The authors feel that such a program could be carried out on a large-scale community basis with a simpler check-up procedure and with a moderate input of resources[25].

In 1986, 110 660 men and women from 33 healthcare clinics in the city of Da Qing, China, were screened for IGT and type 2 diabetes. Of these individuals, 577 were classified (using WHO criteria) as having IGT. Subjects were randomized by clinic into a clinical trial, either to a control group or to one of three active therapy groups: diet only, exercise only, or diet plus exercise. Follow-up evaluations were conducted at 2-year intervals over a 6-year period to identify subjects who developed type 2 diabetes. Cox's proportional hazard analysis was used to determine if the incidence of diabetes varied with the treatment used. The cumulative incidence of diabetes at 6 years was 67.7% in the control group, compared with 43.8% in the diet group, 41.1% in the exercise group and 46% in the diet-plus-exercise group. When analyzed by clinic, each of the active intervention groups differed significantly from the controls. The relative reduction of diabetes development in the active treatment groups was similar when the patients were classified as lean or overweight. In a proportional hazards analysis adjusted for differences in baseline BMI and fasting glucose, the diet, exercise and diet-plus-exercise interventions were associated with 31%, 46% and 42% reduction in risk of developing diabetes respectively. The authors of this study arrived at the conclusion that diet and exercise interventions led to a significant decrease in the incidence of type 2 diabetes over a 6-year period among those with IGT[26].

The Diabetes Prevention Program (DPP), launched in 1996 in the USA, is a 6-year, multicenter trial sponsored by the National Institutes of Health (150 million dollars)[27-30]. The DPP was designed to study a subset of individuals with IGT whose yearly risk of developing diabetes is 7.5% and who have a fasting blood glucose of 100–139 mg/dl; there is over-sampling of individuals from minorities at increased risk. Twenty-five centers were selected to participate in this program. The organizers project that there will be a need to screen between 66 000 and 186 000 people. Of this group, 22 000–47 000 will have IGT with a 25–33% frequency of positive OGTT and of this number 25–33% are expected to satisfy the stricter OGTT requirements of the DPP, leaving 7000–12 000 subjects in the study. Of these, 33–55% would complete the "run-in" phase—a total of 3900 who would ultimately be randomly assigned to different groups[27]. Three study interventions were selected based on their potential efficacy in ameliorating abnormal glucose metabolism in IGT, their safety and tolerable profile of side-effects. The interventions include intensive lifestyle intervention, which focuses on a healthy diet to achieve and maintain at least a 7% loss of body weight and an increase in caloric expenditure of at least 700 kilocalories per week. The drug therapy interventions include metformin and troglitazone. Standard lifestyle recommendations (conventional instructions regarding diet and exercise) will be provided to all participants, including a placebo-treated group which will serve as the control group. After randomization, participants will undergo quarterly evaluations and in addition, a fasting plasma glucose at semi-annual visits and a 75 g OGTT at annual visits. All participants will be followed for 3 years after the closing date for recruitment resulting in 3–6 years of participant follow up. The primary outcome is the development of type 2 diabetes according to WHO criteria. Secondary outcome will focus on cardiovascular disease and its risk factors, change in glycemia, insulin secretion and sensitivity, obesity, physical activity and nutrient intake, quality of life and the occurrence of adverse events[29].

The Diabetes Prevention Study (DPS) is being carried out in Finland, a country with the highest prevalence of diabetes in elderly people. The DPS is a randomized multicenter trial of lifestyle intervention for IGT, aimed at reducing diabetes incidence in this group from 28% to 20%, a change similar to the 40% decrease attained in the Da Qing IGT intervention study. The plan is to treat patients aged 40–64 years who have IGT confirmed on two occasions, whose 2-hour blood glucose level is between 7.8 and 11.0 mmol/l and who have BMI $\geq$ 25. The projected sample size is 530[27].

The Early Diabetes Intervention Trial[31,32] involves 668 self-referred subjects, 46% with normal glucose tolerance, 37% with IGT and 17% with type 2 diabetes. They were randomly assigned to receive acarbose, metformin, both or neither, with a 3-year study planned to assess the effect of these agents on glycemia.

The STOP-NIDDM Trial is an international study on the efficacy of acarbose in preventing or delaying the development of type 2 diabetes in an IGT population[33]. Many studies have been carried out in different countries aimed at determining to what extent and with what methods the progression from IGT to overt type 2 diabetes could be slowed or prevented[34–38].

The intervention studies in IGT present a series of controversial aspects. Earlier trials had serious weaknesses in design and conduct. The major problem in interpreting results from early intervention studies is compliance with the interventions[2]. Gafni[39] tried to assess whether it is possible to perform economic evaluation of a primary prevention strategy in subjects with IGT or whether such a strategy is, for the moment, a "phantom alternative". Unfortunately, the evidence supporting the effectiveness of primary prevention type interventions is weak at best. It is not surprising that no one has suggested a comprehensive strategy (i.e. who is doing what, to whom, where and how often) for an intervention for subjects with IGT. The absence of good evidence about the effectiveness of different IGT intervention precludes a valid economic analysis. "What-if (?)" or "modeling" type studies are likely to result in the typical answer "it depends". It is recommended, therefore, that an economic evaluation should be performed in conjunction with a clinical trial to determine the effectiveness of different IGT interventions[39].

6.3 COMBATING OBESITY AND NUTRITIONAL ERRORS

Bearing in mind the close connection between obesity and type 2 diabetes, the prevention of type 2 diabetes must be based to a large extent on weight control. This aspect has been known since 1921[40]. Unfortunately, medical practice shows that weight loss is notoriously difficult to achieve in obese subjects[41] and the extent to which the abdominal distribution of fat is reversible remains unclear[2]. The problem is more complicated if we take into consideration that metabolically obese but normal-weight individuals are very common in the general population and that they probably represent one end of the spectrum of people with the insulin resistance syndrome[42].

Okauchi *et al.* attempted to evaluate the effectiveness of caloric restriction in preventing the development of diabetes in a model rat (Otsuka Long Evans Tokushima Fatty—OLETF) with type 2 diabetes[43]. Groups of eight male OLETF rats aged 5 weeks were supplied with rat chow *ad libitum* (100% group) and 85% and 70% of the amount of food consumed by the 100% group (85% and 70% groups respectively). The average weights of the three groups were 617, 536 and 450 g at 19 weeks of age and their abdominal fat deposits were 50, 38 and 21 g respectively at 22 weeks of age. At 20 weeks of age, the cumulative incidences of diabetes in the 100%, 85% and 70% groups were 67%, 13% and 0% respectively. The plasma immuno-reactive insulin levels 60 and 120 minutes after oral glucose admin-istration were significantly lower in the 70% group than in the other groups. *In vivo* insulin-stimulated glucose uptake, measured by a euglycemic clamp technique, was significantly higher in the 70% group than in the 100% group. There was no significant difference in the levels of skeletal muscle glucose transporter 4 (GLUT 4) protein. Morphological studies of the pancreas in the 100% group showed enlarged multilobulated fibrotic islets whereas sections of islets in the other groups appeared normal, though slightly enlarged. The results demonstrated that caloric restriction is effective in preventing type 2 diabetes in diabetes-prone rats, probably due to increased insulin sensitivity[43].

In the USA Nurses' Health Study, 2204 cases of type 2 diabetes were diagnosed in 1976–1990 with 1.49 million person-years of follow up[44]. The age-adjusted risk of type 2 diabetes increased linearly across the entire baseline BMI distribution. Compared with women with a BMI < 22.0 kg/m^2, women with a BMI > 34.9 kg/m^2 had a 93.2-fold higher risk of becoming diabetic. Weight gain of even 7–10.9 kg after the age of 18 years was associated with a doubling in the risk of developing type 2 diabetes, whereas a weight loss of more than 5 kg reduced the risk by 50% or more. This study clearly demonstrated the potential for the prevention of type 2 diabetes through effective weight control[2].

Comprehensive programs aimed at combating and preventing obesity have a strong impact in communities in which major lifestyle changes have caused frequency of obesity to grow along with that of type 2 diabetes mellitus. Most studies, for example, of Native American infants, preschool and school-age children and adults have confirmed a high prevalence of excessive weight. Historical studies suggest that for many Native American communities, the high rates of obesity are a relatively recent phenomenon. The specific reasons for this increase have not been discovered, and community-based interventions to modify diet and physical activity in order to prevent obesity and a tendency towards diabetes are needed. Preliminary evidence suggests that these communities are receptive to school-based interventions and that such programs may be able to slow the rate of excessive weight gain and to improve fitness in schoolchildren. As a result of the cultural diversity among Native Americans, future studies should focus on collecting community- and region-specific data and emphasize the need for obesity prevention through culturally appropriate community- and school-based behavioral interventions[45].

The PATHWAYS weight loss program was designed specifically for African-American women, a group with a high frequency of obesity. This program was administered in urban churches by trained lay facilitators and was effective in producing significant and clinically meaningful weight loss. Ongoing research is focusing on whether the results can be maintained or enhanced through monthly reinforcement sessions[46].

An interesting idea originates from a study carried out recently in India[47]. Although the rate and degree of obesity are relatively low among Indians, it has been observed in several investigations that even a minor increase in body mass index increases the risk of developing diabetes. Measures to control weight help to delay the onset of diabetes even in the non-obese, despite a strong family history of the disorder.

As well as a hypocaloric diet, certain drugs—for example orlistat—may delay the onset of type 2 diabetes in high-risk obese patients[48].

One might expect subjects at high risk for development of type 2 diabetes to be highly motivated to lose weight in order to protect their health[49]. However, it has been suggested that the *perception* of risk, rather than *actual* risk, will determine whether an individual will take steps to lower this risk. For instance, individuals who are unaware of their risk or deny their risk would not be expected to take preventive action. Polley *et al.* have observed that perceived risk of developing diabetes and other health beliefs did not predict performance in a behavioral weight loss program. The data of the study suggest that efforts to modify health beliefs by educating high-risk individuals about their risk and the benefits of weight loss may not be effective in improving long-term weight loss. Further research is needed to examine what factors will increase the likelihood that high-risk subjects will take preventive action to reduce their risk[49].

The prophylactic role of diet was conceived mainly as a reduction in calories, total fat and saturated fat and their replacement with complex carbohydrate. Nutritional studies have analyzed (and are still analyzing) the influence of some components of food in the prevention of type 2 diabetes; the results are sometimes controversial[2]. It was suggested long ago that food rich in fiber is a protective factor against diabetes[50] (it is well known that type 2 diabetes is rare in populations living on a diet which is rich in complex carbohydrates and fiber). Recently, an extended follow up of the Nurses' Health Study showed that the risk of developing diabetes in those in the highest quintile of fiber intake (24 g/day) was 0.78 times that in those in the lowest quintile (12 g/day; $p = 0.02$)[51,52]. The preventive approach promoting the use of high-fiber diets in groups at high risk for the development of diabetes is well established. Natural food rich in polysaccharides and fiber such as wholemeal bread, fruits and vegetables should be preferred[2].

6.4 PROMOTION OF PHYSICAL EXERCISE

A gradual decrease in energy output for adults in Western countries has been observed throughout the twentieth century. Based on national survey data, 56% of men and 61% of women in the United States either never or only irregularly engaged in physical activity[53]. Unfortunately, this trend is being increasingly seen[54-56]. The sedentary lifestyle has injurious effects on health and especially increases the risk of cardiovascular disease[54]. The correlation between the development of diabetes and the level of physical activity is being investigated in increasing detail[57]. Numerous studies have consistently shown that higher levels of physical activity are associated with decreased risks of coronary heart disease, cerebrovascular disease, hypertension, type 2 diabetes, colonic and possibly breast cancer, and osteoporosis. The data from these studies indicate that physical activity is effective in prolonging life. Public health professionals worldwide should emphasize the need to increase activity levels during leisure time and to incorporate physical exercise into the daily routine[55]. From the scientific point of view, it is crucial to promote research into the fundamental mechanisms which explain the beneficial effects of physical training on the prevention and the treatment of several diseases[54].

Regular physical activity should be a major goal in the treatment and primary prevention of diabetes[53]. It is thought that increased physical activity delays the onset of type 2 diabetes mellitus or even prevents the disease in about 50% of susceptible individuals (positive family history of type 2 diabetes, body mass index >25, hypertension or gestational diabetes)[58]. The molecular basis of the effects of physical activity on glucose tolerance in diabetics is fairly well understood today. In a manner similar to that of insulin, a single bout of exercise increases the rate of glucose uptake into the contracting skeletal muscles, a process that is regulated by the translocation of GLUT 4 glucose transporters to the plasma membrane and transverse tubules. Exercise and insulin utilize different signaling pathways, both of which lead to the activation of glucose transport, which perhaps explains why individuals with insulin resistance increase muscle glucose transport in response to an acute bout of exercise. Physical training in humans results in numerous beneficial adaptations in the skeletal muscles, including an increase in GLUT 4 expression. The increase in muscle GLUT 4 contributes to an increase in the responsiveness of muscle glucose uptake to insulin, although not all studies show that exercise training in patients with diabetes improves overall glucose control[59].

Changes in muscle morphology as a result of training may also be important in preventing diabetes. With increase in exercise training there is a conversion of fast-twitch glycolytic IIb fibers to fast-twitch oxidative IIa fibers and an increase in capillary density. The IIa fibers have a greater capillary density and are more insulin sensitive and insulin responsive than IIb fibers. Morphological changes in muscle, particularly the capillary density of the muscle, are associated with changes in fasting insulin levels and glucose tolerance. Furthermore, significant correlations between glucose clearance, muscle capillary density and fiber type have been found in humans during a euglycemic clamp. Exercise training may also improve control over hepatic glucose production[60].

Experimental diabetology has produced some interesting data in this field. Exercise training has been shown to be effective in preventing type 2 diabetes in the OLETF rat model mentioned earlier[43]. In order to determine the duration of the preventive effect of exercise training against the development of diabetes in this model, six male OLETF rats each were assigned to training (1) for a whole experimental period from 7 to 28 weeks of age (E-E); (2) for the first half of the period from 7 to 15 weeks of age (E-S); (3) for the second half of the period from 16 to 28 weeks of age (S-E). In addition, eight male OLETF rats were given no exercise during the experimental period (S-S). At 28 weeks of age, E-E, E-S, S-E and S-S rats were weighed: average weights were 514, 542, 557 and 669 g and abdominal fat deposits 13.9, 21.3, 38.2 and 76.0 g respectively. At 28 weeks of age, the cumulative incidence of diabetes in S-S was 100% while none of the trained rats was diabetic. The glucose infusion rate during a hyperinsulinemic euglycemic clamp test, an index of insulin sensitivity, was in the E-E group significantly greater than that in the S-S group. The values in the E-S and S-E groups were slightly, but not significantly, less than that in the E-E group. Morphologic studies on the pancreas of E-E rats and S-E rats showed minimal changes of islets whereas sections of islets from E-S rats appeared slightly enlarged and fibrotic, although significantly less so than those of the islets of S-S rats. These data show that the preventive effect of exercise training against the development of type 2 diabetes lasts for at least 3 months after the cessation of exercise in this animal model[61].

The onset of glucose intolerance could be stopped by maintaining traditional physical activities in certain population groups[62]. In a paper published recently, it was confirmed that regular physical activity plays an important role in the prevention and treatment of human type 2 diabetes[63]. Since physical activity has been shown in prospective studies to protect against the development of type 2 diabetes, physical training programs suitable for individuals at risk for diabetes should be incorporated into the medical care system to a greater extent. One general determinant in a strategy to develop a prevention project for type 2 diabetes is to establish a testing program which includes $VO_{2(max)}$ determinations for individuals who are at risk of developing the disease.

6.4.1 Prospective Studies on the Preventive Role of Physical Exercise in Diabetes

Women aged 21–80 years were interviewed about diabetes; the former athletes were less likely to have diabetes. In those questioned aged over 40 years, the women who had not been college athletes had an age-adjusted rate of diabetes 3.4 times that of the former athletes[64]. A long-term study of the development of chronic disease in former college students demonstrated that there is an inverse correlation between energy expenditure in leisure-time physical activity and the development of type 2 diabetes during the next 14 years[10].

A 2-year follow-up study on a random sample of a population from Malta[65] comprising 388 individuals, classified into three categories of physical activity and three categories of glucose tolerance, showed that baseline physical activity was inversely related to the 2-hour post-challenge blood glucose. In a multivariate analysis, age, family history of diabetes and physical inactivity were the most important predictors of 2-hour blood glucose. The age-standardized risk of glucose intolerance (IGT or type 2 diabetes) was inversely related to the level of physical activity. Among subjects with normal baseline glucose tolerance, those with low physical activity had a risk of glucose intolerance 2.7 times higher at follow up than those with higher physical activity. The results suggested that the protective effect of physical exercise was not confounded by obesity, family history of diabetes or gender[2].

The Nurses' Health Study in the USA involved 87 253 women aged 34–59 years without diabetes at baseline[66]. During 8 years of follow up, 1303 cases of self-reported type 2 diabetes developed. Women who practiced vigorous exercise at least once weekly, had an age-adjusted relative risk (RR) for type 2 diabetes of 0.67 ($p < 0.0001$) compared with women who did not exercise weekly. After adjustment for BMI, the reduction in risk was attenuated but remained significant (RR = 0.84, $p = 0.005$). When the analysis was restricted to the first 2 years after commencing physical activity and to symptomatic type 2 diabetes as the outcome, the age-adjusted RR of those who exercised was 0.5 and age- and BMI-adjusted RR 0.69. Multivariate adjustments for age, BMI, family history of diabetes and other variables did not alter the reduced risk found with exercise[2].

Another important study took into consideration a prospective cohort of 21 271 US male physicians aged 40–48 years during a 5-year follow up[67]. At baseline, information was obtained about the frequency of vigorous exercise and other risk indicators. Over the course of a 105 141-person-years follow-up period, 285 new cases of type 2 diabetes were registered. The age-adjusted incidence of diabetes ranged from 369 cases per 100 000 person-years in subjects who engaged in vigorous exercise less than once weekly to 214 cases per 100 000 person-years in those exercising at least five times per week. Men who exercised at least once per week had an age-adjusted RR of type 2 diabetes of 0.64 compared with those who exercised less frequently. The age-adjusted RR of diabetes decreased with increasing frequency of exercise. A significant decrease in risk persisted after adjustment for both age and BMI. The inverse correlation of type 2 diabetes was particularly pronounced among overweight subjects[2].

In the Honolulu Heart Program, the risk of type 2 diabetes was found to be inversely related to the level of physical activity during a 2- to 6-year follow up of 6815 Japanese-American men aged 45–68 years. There was a dose–response relationship: the greater the level of physical activity, the lower the incidence of type 2 diabetes[68].

The purpose of a more recent study published by Lynch *et al.* was to examine prospectively the association between self-reported levels of the intensity and duration of physical activity, cardiorespiratory fitness (assessed by respiratory gas exchange) and incidence of type 2 diabetes (assessed by the OGTT) in a population-based sample of 897 middle-aged Finnish men. After adjustment for age, baseline glucose values, BMI, serum triglyceride levels, family history of diabetes and alcohol consumption, moderately intense physical activities (≥ 5.5 metabolic units) for at least 40 minutes per week were associated with a reduced risk of type 2 diabetes. Activities with an intensity less than 5.5 metabolic units, regardless of their duration, were not protective. Cardiovascular fitness levels greater than 31.0 ml oxygen per kg per minute were protective against type 2 diabetes. A subgroup of men at high risk for diabetes (because they were overweight and hypertensive and had a positive parental history of the disease), who engaged in moderately intense physical activities above the 40 minutes per week duration reduced their risk by 64% compared with men who did not participate in such activities. Therefore, after adjustment for age, baseline glucose levels and known risk factors, physical activity at an intensity of 5.5 metabolic units or greater and lasting 40 minutes or more per week protected against the development of type 2 diabetes. These protective effects were even more pronounced in a subgroup of men who were at high risk for the development of the disease[69].

The findings from the Pitt County Study suggest that regular physical activity (especially moderate activity) may be associated with a 50–60% reduction in risk for type 2 diabetes in middle-aged African Americans[70].

Examples of what is considered moderate physical activity, taken from the Report of the US Surgeon General (1996) are presented in Table 6.3.

Table 6.3. Examples of moderate amounts of physical activity (defined as activity that burns approximately 150 kilocalories of energy per day or 1000 kilocalories per week)

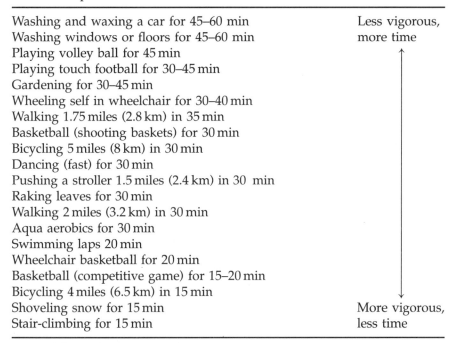

Washing and waxing a car for 45–60 min	Less vigorous,
Washing windows or floors for 45–60 min	more time
Playing volley ball for 45 min	
Playing touch football for 30–45 min	
Gardening for 30–45 min	
Wheeling self in wheelchair for 30–40 min	
Walking 1.75 miles (2.8 km) in 35 min	
Basketball (shooting baskets) for 30 min	
Bicycling 5 miles (8 km) in 30 min	
Dancing (fast) for 30 min	
Pushing a stroller 1.5 miles (2.4 km) in 30 min	
Raking leaves for 30 min	
Walking 2 miles (3.2 km) in 30 min	
Aqua aerobics for 30 min	
Swimming laps 20 min	
Wheelchair basketball for 20 min	
Basketball (competitive game) for 15–20 min	
Bicycling 4 miles (6.5 km) in 15 min	
Shoveling snow for 15 min	More vigorous,
Stair-climbing for 15 min	less time

Adapted from references 71 and 72

The results of all of these studies strongly support the position that people at increased risk for developing type 2 diabetes should be encouraged to maintain a high level of physical activity in their daily lives[2]. In fact, the prophylactic value of physical effort has been proven for numerous pathogenic conditions[73,74].

6.5 IMPROVING LIFESTYLE

Combating obesity and sedentary living means, in the final analysis, an improvement in lifestyle. There are, however, programs and studies that tackle the problem of lifestyle in a global manner[75-79].

Uusitupa[76] states that it is important to carry out long-term controlled studies to find out the extent to which lifestyle modifications could improve the metabolic control and level of major cardiovascular risk factors known to be associated with poor outcome in type 2 diabetes. One-year dietary and exercise intervention on newly diagnosed type 2 diabetic persons in Kuopio, Finland, resulted in better metabolic control and a moderate decrease in cardiovascular risk factors compared with the conventional treatment group. After the second year of follow-up only 12.5% in the intervention group were receiving oral antidiabetic drugs (compared with 34.8% in the conventional treatment group). Weight reduction and a reduced use of saturated fats appeared to be the main determinants of successful treatment results. Good aerobic capacity was associated with an increase in HDL cholesterol. A multicenter primary prevention study on IGT patients is continuing in Finland, applying the same principles of intervention as used in the study on newly diagnosed diabetic patients. Pilot results show that glucose tolerance can be improved by lifestyle changes[76].

The Community Diabetes Prevention Project characterized a population at risk for type 2 diabetes before development of the complete insulin resistance syndrome and is attempting to use lifestyle interventions to alter this progression. Using a diabetes risk assessment tool, the authors identified 412 people (321 women, 91 men; mean age 46 ± 9.8 years). After a baseline evaluation, they were randomized into a standard and an intervention group. The intervention group received an annual assessment with feedback, quarterly newsletters, behavior change program and monthly phone calls for motivation to change diet, exercise and stress behavior. This study is defining the natural history of the development of the insulin resistance syndrome and whether lifestyle interventions over 5 years can prevent the progression to type 2 diabetes[77].

The purpose of another pilot study was to develop an age and culturally appropriate primary intervention program for Mexican-American children of type 2 diabetics. The sample included 37 Mexican-American children aged 7–12 years who had at least one parent or grandparent with type 2 diabetes. A health screen of physiological risk factors, a nutritional assessment and a diabetes knowledge test were administered before and after the program. The eight-session activity-oriented educational program focused on nutrition, exercise and diabetes knowledge. Owing to small sample size and limited study time, changes in physiological factors and diet were not analyzed for statistical significance. Analysis of individual factors showed a trend toward more normal values. Results of this pilot program indicated that health intervention projects may be effective in helping children at risk for type 2 diabetes adopt healthier lifestyles[78].

The prevention of type 2 diabetes mellitus should commence in childhood, especially in populations in which there has been an alarming increase in the frequency of occurrence of this disease. Unfortunately, the prevalence of type 2 diabetes, even in children, has been noted in Pima Indians[80]. Changes in lifestyle in this kind of situation are of capital importance.

6.6   COMBATING OTHER DIABETOGENIC FACTORS

For a pregnant woman found to have glucose intolerance, the high risk of later development of diabetes renders preventive intervention vitally important[12]. Firstly, effective treatment of gestational diabetes is necessary during pregnancy. After pregnancy, dietary intervention should be undertaken to prevent obesity and the women encouraged to take physical exercise. Repeated pregnancy, which increases the risk of diabetes, should be discouraged. Gestational diabetes in the mother may increase the risk of the offspring for developing diabetes, as has been confirmed in Pima Indians[80].

Several states of physical stress or trauma are associated with glucose intolerance induced by hormonal effects on glucose metabolism and insulin secretion or action[12]. The role of emotional and social stress as contributory factors in type 2 diabetes still requires rigorous scientific proof. Nevertheless, these forms of stress are a component of "modern lifestyle" and combating them should not be neglected in the policy of preventing diabetes[77].

There is a long list of medicines and other substances that impair glucose metabolism. Among these are corticosteroids, diuretics of the thiazide type, beta-adrenoreceptor-blocking agents and some contraceptive steroids. They may cause glucose intolerance and, in susceptible subjects, may induce diabetes. This usually resolves after withdrawal of the culprit drug[12]. It is necessary, as a preventive measure, to avoid these products in individuals who have risk factors for type 2 diabetes.

6.7   NEW APPROACHES TO THE PROBLEM

Large-scale screening for potentially diabetic individuals raises important practical and logistic problems[2,39,81]. The OGTT is relatively complex and time-consuming and has poor reproducibility. Measuring fasting plasma glucose (FPG) is a simpler alternative that provides an inexpensive and reproducible glycemic index in non-diabetic and diet-treated diabetic subjects[82]. The Fasting Hyperglycaemia Study Group defined increased fasting glucose (IFG) as a plasma glucose level of at least 5.5 mmol/l but less than 7.8 mmol/l (WHO fasting criteria for diabetes). An initial report from this group describes the identification of subjects with IFG on two consecutive FPG measurements 2 weeks apart for inclusion in the study, which is a randomized intervention trial designed to determine whether progression to diabetes can be delayed or prevented[81]. The study stages are presented in Table 6.4.

Individuals at risk for developing type 2 diabetes were encouraged via a public awareness campaign, general practitioners or direct approach to attend one of three English and two French centers for FPG measurement. Of 1580 subjects (mean age 47 ± 10 years), 29% were men, 56% had a diabetic relative, 20% had a history of elevated glycemia or glycosuria and 9% previously had gestational diabetes.

Table 6.4. Stages in the Fasting Hyperglycaemia Study

I. Subject identification and recruitment for a non-insulin-dependent diabetes trial

II. Randomized controlled trial of reinforced healthy-living advice in subjects with increased but not diabetic fasting plasma glucose

III. Randomized controlled trial of sulfonylurea therapy in subjects with increased but not diabetic fasting plasma glucose

---

Adapted from references 81, 83 and 84

Normal glucose values (i.e. <5.5 mmol/l), were seen in 1046 subjects (66%), 493 (31%) had an initial increased fasting glucose (5.5–7.7 mmol/l) and 41 (3%) a diabetic fasting glucose ($\geq$7.8 mmol/l). Of the 493 with an initial increased fasting glucose, 441 returned for a second FPG measurement and 293 (67%) of those had a similar value 2 weeks later. OGTT in 223 of these subjects showed that 83 (37%) had IGT, 58 (26%) diabetes mellitus and 82 (37%) normal glucose tolerance. While these two glycemic measurements provided good discrimination for diabetes, neither was reliable in detecting those with increased but not diabetic FPG values. Finally, 293 (19%) of the 1580 self-referred subjects were identified as having persistently increased FPG and 227 have been admitted into the prevention trial[81].

These 227 subjects were randomized to reinforced or basic healthy-living advice[83]. They were simultaneously allocated to either a sulfonylurea-receiving group or a control group in a two-by-two factorial design. In three English and two French centers, 201 subjects completed a 1-year follow-up study. Reinforced advice recommending dietary modification and increased exercise was given every 3 months and basic advice was given once at the initial visit. Glycemia was monitored by FPG, dietary compliance by body weight and food diaries and fitness compliance by bicycle ergometer assessment and exercise diaries. Both reinforced and basic advice groups had a significant decrease in body weight (1.5 kg) at 3 months, although the weight subsequently returned to baseline. After 1 year, subjects allotted to reinforcement advice versus basic advice (1) reported a lower fat intake with no difference in lipid profiles, (2) had improved fitness, as demonstrated by increased calculated maximal oxygen uptake with no change in insulin sensitivity, (3) showed no change in FPG, glucose tolerance or hemoglobin A1c and (4) showed a greater tendency to withdraw from the study. After this phase of the study, the authors came to the conclusion that reinforced healthy living advice given to self-referred subjects with increased FPG did not encourage sufficiently pronounced lifestyle changes to have significantly greater effects on body weight and glycemia than basic healthy living advice. As diabetes is a chronic progressive disease, a longer period of reinforced healthy living advice is necessary in Western societies to determine the possible advantages[83].

Subjects were also randomized to sulfonylurea therapy (glicazide ≤160 mg/day) or to a control group taking either placebo or no tablets[84]. Those allotted to glicazide had a significant reduction in median FPG compared with the control group. Median hemoglobin A1c also improved, as did mean beta-cell fuction. Mean body weight was unchanged in the glicazide group, but decreased in the control group. More subjects in the glicazide than the control group reported one or more minor symptoms of hypoglycemia over 1 year. Only two subjects reported major hypoglycemic episodes requiring assistance, both of whom were taking glicazide. Insulin sensitivity did not change between groups. Sulfonylurea treatment using glicazide improved glycemic control and beta-cell function significantly in subjects with increased but not diabetic FPG levels. The study is being extended to 6 years follow up to determine whether sulfonylurea therapy prevents progression to type 2 diabetes[84].

6.8 PARTICULAR ASPECTS

An attempt at systematization of the problems raised by the prevention of type 2 diabetes mellitus cannot be concluded without commenting on some particular aspects, even if some of these have been mentioned in passing in previous pages (Table 6.5).

One of the most debated issues is that of communities and populations in which diabetes attains high frequencies, usually as a result of changes from the traditional lifestyle. Daniel and Gamble confirm that the high prevalence of diabetes in Canada's native communities corresponds with the high prevalence rates in other populations of indigenous peoples that have experienced the changes associated with acculturation. Behavioral risk factors can be

Table 6.5. Some aspects of special interest in the prevention of type 2 diabetes

Population and communities with a high frequency of type 2 diabetes
Preventive measures in children and adolescents
The major role of education
The major role of primary healthcare providers
The church could make a notable contribution

particularly amenable to public health campaigns. There is a need to develop, implement and test in cooperation with native people interventions aimed at reducing the frequency and consequences of type 2 diabetes by reducing the risk of its onset and by early detection and treatment. Intervention programs should be developed with attention being paid to the overall health, social, economic, educational and cultural environment within a community[85].

American Indians and Alaska natives have also experienced rapidly increasing rates of type 2 diabetes[1,14,15,19,80,86]. To address this epidemic Indian Health Service (HIS) and tribal communities have developed primary, secondary and tertiary intervention strategies. The scientific basis for secondary and tertiary prevention supports well-defined care practices, and surveillance of the implementation of these practices (as well as their influence on metabolic and hypertension control as a standard community intervention for the primary prevention of diabetes) is under way, reflecting the priorities of individual communities[86].

The project designated DIRECT (Diabetes Intervention Reaching and Educating Communities Together) is a multilevel community-based intervention project designed to address diabetes and its complications. Diabetes mellitus is a major public health problem in the African-American community of Wake county, North Carolina. Modifiable risk factors for diabetes and undiagnosed diabetes are common. Project DIRECT is attempting to improve the health-related quality of life of this population by reducing the burden of diabetes and its complications[87].

An aspect closely connected to the above is that of the preventive measures aimed at children and adolescents. For example, the incidence of type 2 diabetes has increased dramatically in the past decade in Pima children aged 5–17 years, living in the Gila River Indian Community. As a result, a diabetes primary prevention program called Quest was implemented in 1996 at an elementary school in the region for students in kindergarten and grades 1–2. The Quest program has four components: (1) biochemical and anthropometric assessments; (2) classroom instruction about diabetes; (3) increased daily physical activity at school; and (4) a structured school breakfast and lunch program. Preliminary results of this project indicate that the school provides a stable environment for behavior change and interventions that slow weight gain in early childhood[88].

The Zuni Diabetes Prevention Program is another community-based primary prevention project designed to reduce the prevalence of diabetes risk factors among youths in high school. The program strives to enhance knowledge of diabetes and to support physical activity, increased fruit and vegetable intake and reduced soft drink consumption. The primary mechanisms of intervention are diabetes education, a school-based health center, supportive social networks and modification of the food supply available to teens. Program evaluation uses a multiple cross-sectional model. Assessment occurs at three points within the 4-year project. Mid-project results indicated a significant reduction in soft drink consumption and an increase in glucose/insulin ratios, suggesting a decline in the incidence of hyperglycemia[89].

Optimization of lifestyle factors by quitting smoking, losing weight, proper nutrition and starting an exercise regimen is the cornerstone of treatment for dyslipidemias, diabetes and heart disease. However, any healthcare practitioner who has recommended lifestyle changes to a patient knows the inherent difficulty for most patients who try to implement and adhere to such behavior changes. For this reason, it must be emphasized that patient education is a fundamental component of comprehensive clinical care and is a necessary antecedent to behavior change[90]. Through effective education, patients can learn prevention strategies, reduce their risk status and make better lifestyle choices in order to optimize their health and well-being. Providing patient education, however, can be a complex task and requires healthcare practitioners to go beyond simply telling the patient what to do. How can healthcare providers be more efficient in their teaching efforts? Integrating key theoretical perspectives on patient education and using a sound, consistent approach in teaching patients will improve the efficacy of education and ensure more proficient implementation of this role in the context of medical practice. Taking "AIM" is one such approach—Assess the learner, Identify barriers to learning and Motivate the patient to make changes[90].

The decisive role of medical personnel at all levels, especially that of primary care providers, must be highlighted. The physiologic mechanism involved in development of the preliminary phase of type 2 diabetes or X syndrome is particularly amenable to primary and secondary prevention and to health promotion activities. Nurse Practitioners provide an alternative delivery of care based on health promotion and disease prevention principles. Working in a primary delivery model with individuals at risk for diabetes nurse practitioners have the opportunity to bring about measurable outcome differences[91].

The possible contribution of the church has been discussed[46]. Recently, Simmons *et al.* studied the impact of a 2-year pilot church-based diabetes risk reduction program on major lifestyle predictors for type 2 diabetes (exercise and weight control) in a prospective, non-randomized controlled study of a modular lifestyle and diabetes awareness intervention program using a community development model. The study involved two complete church congregations from an ethnic group at high risk of diabetes (Western Samoans) (intervention church $n = 78$; control church $n = 144$). Weight remained stable in the intervention church but increased in the control church. In the intervention church, there was an associated reduction in waist circumference, increase in diabetes knowledge and an increase in the proportion of regular exercise. Consumption of key fatty foods was also reduced. The authors concluded that diabetes risk reduction programs based upon lifestyle change, diabetes awareness and empowerment of high-risk communities can significantly reduce risk factors for future type 2 diabetes[92].

It can be presumed that not just churches and schools but other important components of contemporary human society will be gradually attracted to the prevention of diabetes and other major diseases.

NOTE ADDED AT PROOF

The Diabetes Prevention Program (DPP) was recently redefined[93]. It is a randomized clinical trial for testing strategies to prevent or delay the development of type 2 diabetes in high-risk individuals with elevated fasting plasma glucose concentrations or IGT. Twenty seven clinical centers in the USA are recruiting at least 3000 participants, to be assigned at random to one of three intervention groups: an intensive lifestyle intervention (healthy diet and exercise) and two masked medication treatment groups – metformin or placebo – combined with standard diet and excercise. A fourth treatment group – troglitazone combined with standard diet and excercise – was included initially but discontinued because of the liver toxicity of the drug[93].

REFERENCES

1. Bennet PH, Knowler WC. Early detection and intervention in diabetes mellitus: is it effective? *J Chron Dis* 1984; **37**: 653–666.
2. Tuomilehto J, Tuomilehto-Wolf E, Zimmet P, Alberti KGMM, Knowler WC. Primary prevention of Diabetes Mellitus. In Alberti KGMM, Zimmet P, DeFronzo RA, Keen H (eds). *International Textbook of Diabetes Mellitus*, 2nd edn. Chichester: Wiley, 1997; 1799–1827.
3. Tuomilehto J, Knowler WC, Zimmet P. Primary prevention of non-insulin-dependent diabetes mellitus. *Diabetes Metab Rev* 1992; **8**: 339–353.
4. Boucher BJ, Ewen SWB, Stowers JM. Betel nut (*Areca catechu*) consumption and the induction of diabetes in adult CD1 mice and their F1 and F2 offspring. *Diabetologia* 1994; **37**: 49–55.
5. Holemans K, Aerts L, van Assche FA. Evidence for an insulin resistance in the adult offspring of pregnant STZ-diabetic rats. *Diabetologia* 1991; **34**: 81–85.
6. Boucher BJ. Strategies for reduction in the prevalence of NIDDM; the case for a population-based approach to the development of policies to deal with environmental factors in its aetiology. *Diabetologia* 1995; **38**: 1125–1129.
7. Henry RR. Prospects for primary prevention of type 2 diabetes mellitus. *Diabetes Rev Int* 1994; **3**: 2–5.
8. Khaw K-T. Genetics and environment: Geoffrey Rose revisited. *Lancet* 1994; **343**: 839–839.
9. Diabetes Epidemiology Research International. Preventing insulin dependent diabetes mellitus: the environmental challenge. *BMJ* 1987; **295**: 479–481.
10. Helmrich SP, Ragland DR, Lueng RW, Paffenbarger RS Jr. Physical activity and reduced occurrence of non-insulin dependent diabetes mellitus. *N Engl J Med* 1991; **325**: 147–152.

11. Trovati M, Carta Q, Cavalot F *et al.* Influence of physical training on blood glucose control, glucose intolerance, insulin secretion and insulin action in non-insulin dependent diabetic patients. *Diabetes Care* 1984; **7**: 416–420.
12. WHO. *Prevention of Diabetes Mellitus. Report of a WHO Study Group.* Geneva: World Health Organization, 1994.
13. Simmons D, Voyle J, Swinburn B, O'Dea K. Community-based approaches for the primary prevention of non-insulin-dependent diabetes mellitus. *Diabetic Med* 1997; **14**: 519–526.
14. Knowler WC, Narayan KM, Hanson RL *et al.* Preventing non-insulin-dependent diabetes. *Diabetes* 1995; **44**: 483–488.
15. Narayan KM, Hanson RL, Pettitt DJ, Bennett PH, Knowler WC. A two-step strategy for identification of high-risk subjects for a clinical trial of the prevention of NIDDM. *Diabetes Care* 1996; **19**: 927–978.
16. Mudaliar SR, Henry RR. Strategies for preventing type II diabetes. What can be done to stem the epidemic? *Postgrad Med* 1997; **102**: 181–186.
17. Fuchs H. The possibility of preventing non-insulin dependent diabetes. *Przegl Lek* 1996; **53**: 668–671.
18. Chausmer AB. Zinc, insulin and diabetes. *J Am Coll Nutr* 1998; **17**: 109–115.
19. Harris MI, Hadden WC, Knowler WC, Bennett PH. Prevalence of diabetes and impaired glucose tolerance and plasma glucose levels in US populations aged 20–74 years. *Diabetes* 1987; **36**: 523–534.
20. Edelstein SL, Knowler WC, Bain RP *et al.* Predictors of progression from impaired glucose tolerance to NIDDM: an analysis of six prospective studies. *Diabetes* 1997; **46**: 701–710.
21. Melander A. Review of previous impaired glucose tolerance intervention studies. *Diabetic Med* 1996; **13** (Suppl 2): 520–522.
22. Jarrett RJ, Keen H, Fuller JH, McCartney P. Worsening to diabetes in men with impaired glucose tolerance ("borderline diabetes"). *Diabetologia* 1979; **16**: 25–30.
23. Keen H, Jarret RJ, McCartney P. Ten-years follow-up of the Bedford survey (1962–1972): glucose tolerance and diabetes. *Diabetologia* 1982; **22**: 73–78.
24. Sartor G, Scherster B, Carlstron S, Melander A, Norden A, Persson G. Ten-year follow-up of subjects with impaired glucose tolerance prevention of diabetes by tolbutamide and diet regulation. *Diabetes* 1980; **29**: 41–49.
25. Eriksson K-F, Lidgärde F. Prevention of Type 2 (non-insulin-dependent) diabetes mellitus by diet and physical exercise. The 6-year Malmö feasibility study. *Diabetologia* 1991; **34**: 891–898.
26. Pan XR, Li GW, Hu YH *et al.* Effects of diet and exercise in preventing

NIDDM in people with impaired glucose tolerance. The Da Qing IGT and Diabetes Study. *Diabetes Care* 1997; **20**: 537–544.

27. Bloomgarden ZT. American Diabetes Association Annual Meeting, 1997. Obesity, diabetes prevention and type 1 diabetes. *Diabetes Care* 1997; **20**: 1913–1917.

28. Linday LA. Trivalent chromium and the diabetes prevention program. *Med Hypotheses* 1997; **49**: 47–49.

29. Florez H. Pasos hacia la prevencion primaria de la diabetes mellitus tipo II. Algunas consideraciones epidemiologicas. *Invest Clin* 1997; **38**: 39–52.

30. Leontos C, Wong F, Gallivan J, Lising M. National Diabetes Education Program: Opportunities and challenges. *J Am Diet Assoc* 1998; **98**: 73–75.

31. Holman R, North B, Tunbridge F on behalf of the EDIT Study Group. Early Diabetes Intervention Trial. *Diabetes* 1997; **46** (Suppl 1): 157A.

32. Holman RR, North BV, Tunbridge FKE on behalf of the EDIT study group. Early Diabetes Intervention Trial. *Diabetologia* 1997; **40** (Suppl 1): A17.

33. Chiasson J-L, Gomis R, Hanefeld M, Josse RG, Karasik A, Laakso M. The STOP-NIDDM Trial. Study to prevent type 2 diabetes. *Diabetologia* 1998; **41** (Suppl 1): A127.

34. Bourn DM. The potential for lifestyle change to influence the progression of impaired glucose tolerance to non-insulin-dependent diabetes mellitus. *Diabetic Med* 1996; **13**: 938–945.

35. Hreidarsson AB, Arnardottir I, Helgason T. Treating impaired glucose tolerance. Long-term results. *Diabetologia* 1998; **41** (Suppl 1): A127.

36. Li JKY, Ko GTC, Chan JCN *et al.* The progression of IGT to NIDDM in Chinese—Is there a role in diet and drug treatment? *Diabetologia* 1997; **40** (Suppl 1): A193.

37. Khamina-Drozdov H. Dynamic observation of patients with impaired glucose tolerance. *Diabetologia* 1997; **40** (Suppl 1): A194.

38. Taylor T. The effect of orlistat on glucose tolerance in obese non-diabetic inidviduals. *Diabetologia* 1997; **40** (Suppl 1): A197.

39. Gafni A. Economic implications of IGT intervention: the case of a "phantom alternative"? *Diabetic Med* 1996; **13** (Suppl 2): S25–28.

40. Joslin EP. The prevention of diabetes mellitus. *JAMA* 1921; **75**: 79–84.

41. National Institutes of Health. Consensus development conference on diet and exercise in non-insulin-dependent diabetes mellitus. *Diabetes Care* 1987; **10**: 639–644.

42. Ruderman N, Chisholm D, Pi-Sunyer X, Schneider S. The metabolically obese, normal-weight individual revisited. *Diabetes* 1998; **47**: 699–713.

43. Okauchi N, Mizuno A, Yoshimoto S, Zhu M, Sano T, Shima K. Is caloric restriction effective in preventing diabetes mellitus in the Otsuka Long Evans Tokushima Fatty rat, a model of spontaneous non-insulin-dependent diabetes mellitus? *Diabetes Res Clin Pract* 1995; **27**: 7–106.

44. Colditz GA, Willett WC, Rotnitzky A, Manson JE. Weight gain as a risk factor for clinical diabetes mellitus in women. *Ann Intern Med* 1995; **122**: 481–486.

45. Broussard BA, Sugarman JR, Bachman-Carter K *et al.* Toward comprehensive obesity prevention programs in Native American communities. *Obesity Res* 1995; **3** (Suppl 2): 289s–297s.

46. McNabb W, Quinn M, Kerver J, Cook S, Karrison T. The PATHWAYS church-based weight loss program for urban African-American women at risk for diabetes. *Diabetes Care* 1997; **20**: 1518–1523.

47. Viswanathan M, Snehalatha C, Viswanathan V, Vidyavathi P, Indu J, Ramachandran A. Reduction in body weight helps to delay the onset of diabetes even in non-obese with strong family history of the disease. *Diabetes Res Clin Pract* 1997: **35**: 107–112.

48. Wilding JPH. Obesity treatment with orlistat (Xenical®) helps to prevent deterioration in glucose tolerance. *Diabetologia* 1998; **41** (Suppl 1): A126.

49. Polley BA, Jakicic JM, Venditti EM, Barr S, Wing RR. The effects of health beliefs on weight loss in individuals at high risk for NIDDM. *Diabetes Care* 1997; **20**: 1533–1538.

50. Trowell H. Diabetes mellitus and dietary fiber of starchy foods. *Am J Clin Nutr* 1978; **31**: 553–557.

51. Salmerón J, Stampfer MJ, Colditz GA, Manson JE, Wing AL, Willett WC. Dietary fiber, glycemic load and risk of non-insulin-dependent diabetes mellitus in women. *JAMA* 1997; **277**: 472–477.

52. Wolever TMS, Hanrad S, Gittelsohn J *et al.* Low dietary fiber and high protein intakes associated with newly diagnosed diabetes in a remote aboriginal community. *Am J Clin Nutr* 1997; **66**: 1470–1474.

53. Spelsberg A, Manson JE. Physical activity in the treatment and prevention diabetes. *Compr Ther* 1995; **21**: 559–562.

54. Rieu M. Role of physical activities in a public health policy. *Bull Acad Natl Med* 1995; **179**: 1417–1426.

55. Lee IM, Pafenberger RS Jr., Hennekens CH. Physical activity, physical fitness and longevity. *Aging (Milano)* 1997; **9**: 2–11.

56. Pereira MA, Kriska AM, Joswiak ML *et al.* Physical inactivity and glucose intolerance in the multiethnic island of Mauritius. *Med Sci Sports Exerc* 1995; **27**: 1626–1634.

57. Eriksson K-F, Lindgärde F. Poor physical fitness and impaired early insulin response but late hyperinsulinaemia, as predictors of NIDDM in middle-aged Swedish men. *Diabetologia* 1996; **39**: 573–579.

58. Lehman R, Spinas GA. Role of physical activity in the therapy and prevention of Type II diabetes mellitus. *Ther Umsch* 1996; **53**: 925–933.

59. Goodyear LJ, Kahn BB. Exercise, glucose transport, and insulin sensitivity. *Annu Rev Med* 1998; **49**: 235–261.

60. Ivy JL. Role of exercise training in the prevention and treatment of insulin resistance and non-insulin-dependent diabetes mellitus. *Sports Med* 1997; **24**: 321–336.
61. Shima K, Shi K, Mizumo A, Sano T, Ishida K, Noma Y. Exercise training has a long-lasting effect on prevention of non-insulin-dependent diabetes mellitus in Otsuka-Long-Evans-Tokushima Fatty rats. *Metabolism* 1996; **45**: 475–480.
62. Adler AI, Boyko EJ, Schraer CD, Murphy NJ. The negative association between traditional physical activities and the prevalence of glucose intolerance in Alaska Natives. *Diabetic Med* 1996; **13**: 555–560.
63. Walberg-Henriksson H, Rincon J, Zierath JR. Exercise in the management of non-insulin-dependent diabetes mellitus. *Sports Med* 1998; **25**: 25–35.
64. Frisch RE, Wyshak G, Albright TE, Albright NL, Schiff I. Lower prevalence of diabetes in female former college athletes compared with non-athletes. *Diabetes* 1986; **35**: 1101–1105.
65. Schranz A, Tuomilehto J, Marti B *et al.* Low physical activity and worsening of glucose tolerance: results from a 2-year follow-up of a population sample in Malta. *Diabetes Res Clin Pract* 1991; **11**: 127–136.
66. Manson JE, Rimm EB, Stampfer MJ *et al.* Physical activity and incidence of non-insulin-dependent diabetes mellitus in women. *Lancet* 1991; **338**: 338–778.
67. Manson JE, Nathan DM, Krolewski AS *et al.* A prospective study of exercise and incidence of diabetes among US male physicians. *JAMA* 1992; **268**: 63–67.
68. Burchfield CM, Sharp DS, Curb JD *et al.* Physical activity and incidence of diabetes: the Honolulu Heart Program. *Am J Epidemiol* 1995; **141**: 360–368.
69. Lynch J, Helmrich SP, Lakka TA *et al.* Moderately intense physical activities and high levels of cardiorespiratory fitness reduce the risk of non-insulin-dependent diabetes mellitus in middle-aged men. *Arch Intern Med* 1996; **156**: 1307–1314.
70. James SA, Jamjoun L, Raghunathan TE, Strogatz DS, Furth ED, Khazamie PG. Physical activity and NIDDM in African-Americans: the Pitt County Study. *Diabetes Care* 1998; **21**: 555–562.
71. *Physical activity and health. A Report of the Surgeon General.* US Department of Health and Human Services, Washington, 1996.
72. Lefèbvre P. Can exercise prevent the occurrence of Type II diabetes mellitus? *Reducing the Burden of Diabetes J* 1998; **12**: 2–4.
73. Jako P. The role of physical activity in the prevention of certain internal diseases. *Orv Hetil* 1995; **136**: 2379–2383.
74. Evans WJ. Effects of exercise on body composition and functional capacity of the elderly. *J Gerontol A Biol Sci Med Sci* 1995; **50**: 147–150.

75. Bourn DM. The potential for lifestyle change to influence the progression of impaired glucose tolerance to non-insulin-dependent diabetes mellitus. *Diabetic Med* 1996; **13**: 938–945.

76. Uusitupa MI. Early lifestyle intervention in patients with non-insulin-dependent diabetes mellitus and impaired glucose tolerance. *Ann Med* 1996; **28**: 445–449.

77. Bergenstal R, Monk A, Leite S, Nelson J, List S, Upham P. The Community Diabetes Prevention Project (CDPP). *Diabetologia* 1997; **40** (Suppl 1): A195.

78. McKenzie SB, O'Connell J, Smith LA, Ottinger WE. A primary intervention program (pilot study) for Mexican American children at risk for type 2 diabetes. *Diabetes Educator* 1998; **24**: 180–187.

79. Wing RR, Vendith B, Jakicic J, Buther B, Dyke S. Lifestyle intervention for obese subjects with a family history of diabetes. *Diabetes* 1995; **44** (Suppl 1): 256A.

80. Dabelea D, Hanson RL, Bennett PH, Roumain J, Knowler WC, Pettitt DJ. Increasing prevalence of Type II diabetes in American Indian children. *Diabetologia* 1998; **41**: 904–910.

81. Hammersley MS, Meyer LC, Morris RJ, Nanley SE, Turner RC, Holman RR. The Fasting Hyperglycaemia Study: I. Subject identification and recruitment for a non-insulin-dependent diabetes prevention trial. *Metabolism* 1997; **46** (Suppl 1): 44–49.

82. Holman RR, Turner RC. The basal plasma glucose: A simple relevant index of diabetes. *Clin Endocrinol* 1981; **14**: 279–286.

83. Dyson PA, Hammersley MS, Morris RJ, Holman RR, Turner RC. The Fasting Hyperglycaemia Study: II. Randomized controlled trial of reinforced healthy-living advice in subjects with increased but not diabetic fasting plasma glucose. *Metabolism* 1997; **46** (Suppl 1): 50–55.

84. Karunakaran S, Hammersley MS, Morris RJ, Turner RC, Holman RR. The Fasting Hyperglycaemia Study: III. Randomized controlled trial of sulfonylurea therapy in subjects with increased but not diabetic fasting plasma glucose. *Metabolism* 1997; **46** (Suppl 1): 56–60.

85. Daniel M, Gamble D. Diabetes and Canada's aboriginal peoples: the need for primary prevention. *Int J Nurs Stud* 1995; **32**: 243–259.

86. Gohdes D, Schraer C, Rith-Najarian S. Diabetes prevention in American Indians and Alaska Natives: where we are in 1994? *Diabetes Res Clin Pract* 1996; **34** (Suppl): S95–S100.

87. Herman WH, Thompson TJ, Visscher W *et al.* Diabetes mellitus and its complications in an African-American community: project DIRECT. *J Natl Med Assoc* 1998; **90**: 147–156.

88. Cook VV, Hurley JS. Prevention of type 2 diabetes in childhood. *Clin Pediatr* 1998; **37**: 123–129.

89. Teufel NI, Ritenbaugh CK. Development of a primary prevention program: insight gained in the Zuni Diabetes Prevention Program. *Clin Pediatr* 1998; **37**: 131–141.
90. Kingsbury K. Taking AIM: how to teach primary and secondary prevention effectively. *Can J Cardiol* 1998; **14** (Suppl A): 22A–26A.
91. Sinsel-Phillips P. Syndrome X. Primary care provider's role in health promotion and disease prevention. *Nurse Pract* 1996; **21**: 66, 69–70.
92. Simmons D, Fleming C, Voyle J, Fou F, Feo S, Gatland B. A pilot urban church-based programme to reduce risk factors for diabetes among Western Samoans in New Zealand. *Diabetic Med* 1998; **15**: 136–142.
93. The Diabetes Prevention Program Research Group. The diabetes prevention program: design and methods for a clinical trial in the prevention of type 2 diabetes. *Diabetes Care* 1999; **22**: 623–634.

7

General Evaluation of the Prophylaxis of Diabetes Mellitus

After the discussion of the theoretical basis and the practical aspects of the prophylaxis of diabetes mellitus at present, the moment for a general evaluation of the problem has come. There will be an attempt in this chapter to present suggestions and more or less original ideas for stimulating interest in the prevention of diabetes mellitus in both medical personnel and other groups of, and forces in, human society.

7.1 AWARENESS OF DANGER

The great number of diabetic individuals and, in particular, the uncontrolled increase in this number has been signaled in periodicals and specialist congresses everywhere. Prestigious medical and scientific organizations (the World Health Organization, International Diabetes Federation, European Association for the Study of Diabetes and the American Diabetes Association amongst others) are more and more insistently drawing attention to the "pandemic of diabetes" and offering detailed data about the unique dimensions and development of the phenomenon. The fact that this sort of information is disseminated so as to increase public awareness of the magnitude of the danger that diabetes mellitus represents is significant. Aside from the general increase in diabetes, other epidemiologic aspects of the disease deserve to be borne in mind—such as the exceptional increase in the incidence of type 2 diabetes, its preferential increase in developing countries and the excessive increase in some segments of the populace whose lifestyle has changed radically.

The statistics and evaluations of the costs of diabetes have been growing in number. Contemporary society has noted, with growing anxiety, the huge sums of money consumed in the care of this disease and there are increasingly strong opinions that efficient prophylaxis is the only reasonable alternative to this immense waste[1].

Nevertheless, we must not delude ourselves. Much time and effort must be expended before the truth about diabetes becomes known in all strata of society of every nation and before strong attitudes to the disease will develop.

7.2 PROGRESS IN THE AREA OF ETIOPATHOGENESIS

Our knowledge about the causes and mechanisms of the genesis of diabetes have increased remarkably, lending support to the need for preventive action.

Both principal types of diabetes develop on a certain genetic basis. This has been better defined in the case of type 1 diabetes and involves MHC and non-MHC genes. However, preventive measures that will include genetic maneuvers are still in the future for human diabetes. The application of gene therapy to type 1 diabetes awaits improvements in gene transfer techniques and the development of better tools for accurate diagnosis of prediabetic people[2].

Amongst the environmental factors involved in the production of type 1 diabetes are viruses (the most suspect at the moment being mumps, Coxsackie B and congenital rubella) and some nutritional agents (such as cows' milk proteins)[3]. For type 2 diabetes, the most important etiologic contributions come from obesity, lack of physical activity and a "modern" lifestyle[4].

The pathogenesis of type 1 diabetes is dominated by autoimmune mechanisms, even if there are cases in which this cannot be demonstrated. Two essential mechanisms have been implicated in the pathogenesis of type 2 diabetes: insulin resistance and insulin secretory dysfunction. In consequence of these, a constant progression from IGT to overt diabetes has been noted.

It could be said, with some accuracy, that the most significant preventive projects for type 1 diabetes aim at influencing some immunologic aspects of this disorder. For type 2 diabetes, preventive efforts concentrate on the main environmental aspects. When these are removed, insulin sensitivity improves and the disease may regress[2].

7.3 PROGRESS IN EXPERIMENTAL DIABETOLOGY

A great and valuable contribution to the development of methods of prevention of type 1 diabetes has been made by the studies of animals, especially of NOD mice and BB rats. These rodents have the advantage of developing a spontaneous autoimmune diabetes very similar to human diabetes. Among their disadvantages, the most important are the deficiency of T lymphocytes (for BB rats) and the predominance of diabetes in females (for NOD mice)[5].

Animal models of type 2 diabetes have also been used in studies of prevention and it is not to be ruled out that, in future, this direction of research will gain in significance.

7.4 PREVENTION OF HUMAN TYPE 1 DIABETES

Some of the methods of prevention attempted in animal diabetes have constituted the take-off point for trials for the prevention of human type 1 diabetes. The greatest hope at the moment lies in nicotinamide, the parenteral administration of insulin and oral antigen tolerization. These means cannot be included in true primary prevention but rather in secondary prevention.

One major approach currently being tested for type 1 diabetes prevention is that of beta-cell protection by using high doses of the B-vitamin nicotinamide[6]. In rodent islet cells, the main target of nicotinamide is the enzyme poly(ADP-ribose) polymerase. This enzyme may deplete the intracellular nicotinamide adenine dinucleotide pool, when activated by DNA strand breaks in damaged beta cells, for the synthesis of poly(ADP-ribose)[7]. Nicotinamide was initially tried for beta-cell protection in type 1 diabetes patients after the onset of the disease. A meta-analysis of 16 published studies failed to demonstrate clinical improvement but found evidence for improved beta-cell function after 1 year of treatment. The results of this meta-analysis support the rationale behind, and safety of, the ongoing large multi-center trials of nicotinamide for the prevention of type 1 diabetes[8]. A few pilot trials in ICA-positive first-degree relatives of patients have been reported but the data are inconsistent[9-11]. A large, non-placebo-controlled but randomized trial in more than 33000 schoolchildren showed a 40% lower rate of diabetes in the nicotinamide-treated group[12]. Two randomized, placebo-controlled multicenter trials have subsequently been initiated[13,14]: The International European Nicotinamide Diabetes Intervention Trial (ENDIT) includes groups from 24 countries—an interim analysis was scheduled for September 1998 and the trial was expected to conclude in 2002[13]; The Deutsche Nicotinamide Intervention Study (DENIS) was carried out by German and Austrian pediatricians[14] and the results were published in June 1998[15]. As Elliot *et al.* have observed, nicotinamide has a protective effect against the development of type 1 diabetes but the size of the effect varies widely. Further follow up may define the magnitude of the protective effect within narrower limits[12].

Prophylactic insulin therapy is based on the idea that insulin is the only target autoantigen identified to date in human type 1 diabetes which is exclusively beta-cell specific. After the first preventive trials with parenteral insulin on human subjects, it appears that a combination of intravenous and subcutaneous insulin would be the most efficient, followed by subcutaneous insulin alone[16]. The protocol of the DPT-1 plans that parenteral insulin be used in first-degree relatives with a greater than 50% projected 5-year risk. The subjects of the intervention will be followed over a period of 5–6 years. The initiators are of the opinion that this trial will serve as a prototype for any future intervention, whether refinements of insulin therapy are being explored or new approaches are being tried[17].

As was demonstrated in Chapter 4, oral antigen tolerization could be considered one of the most interesting and encouraging possibilities for type 1 diabetes prevention. The oral arm of the DPT-1 began in September 1996. Investigators present periodic information about the development of its principal aspects[18]. A European diabetes oral tolerance study has been initiated. This is a multicenter, double-blind, randomized trial of oral tolerance with insulin in double/triple antigen-specific autoantibody-positive, HLA-DQB1*0602-negative first-degree relatives of type 1 diabetes patients. Following revision of the protocol, the proposal to use a mixture of insulin and recombinant CTB for the "treated subjects" was made. The use of CTB may potentiate the induction of oral tolerance without any enhancement in antibody formation[19].

With this remarkable scientific base, the prevention of type 1 diabetes is still far from being realized in practice on a large scale. None of the methods proposed has shown the necessary qualities for this—or, in fact, gone beyond the stage of trials.

7.5   PREVENTION OF TYPE 2 DIABETES MELLITUS

Although at first glance it would appear simple, the prevention of type 2 diabetes is difficult from the theoretical, and especially from the practical, point of view. In all probability, the major obstacle impeding the realization of efficient prophylaxis of this disease is its close connection with the negative aspects of the so-called "modern lifestyle" (obesity, nutritional errors, reduction in physical activity, stress, smoking, alcohol consumption, etc.). This opinion is strongly supported by the observations made on those population groups that have undergone drastic change in their traditional mode of life to the "Western" lifestyle. Many of the prevention projects have just such groups, which are at high risk for diabetes, in mind.

As was mentioned in 1991 by Stern[20], a public health strategy for combating chronic diseases consists of three phases: (1) observational epidemiologic studies; (2) first cross-sectional and then prospective intervention trials; and, finally (3) public health action. By comparison with cardiovascular diseases, public health action (in some areas of the world) in the field of type 2 diabetes is lagging far behind. The author appreciates that numerous trial designs should be considered for testing the hypothesis about the primary prevention of type 2 diabetes. These include single risk factors, multiple risk factors and factorial designs[20].

In Chapter 6, I evaluated several of the trials effected to date or currently in progress. Some have concentrated on combating obesity and nutritional errors. Others have in mind, preferentially, the promotion of physical activity. Achievable reductions in the risk of type 2 diabetes by favorably altering its modifiable determinants were estimated to be 50–75% for obesity and 30–50% for physical activity[21]. Other projects have commenced from a broader approach to the problem of lifestyle.

The intervention studies in IGT have enjoyed special attention. Amongst these are the Malmö feasibility study, the Da Qing IGT and Diabetes Study, the Diabetes Prevention Program (DPP) and other well known and widely commented-upon studies. Bearing in mind the practical and logistic difficulties connected to IGT, we thought it necessary to discuss some simpler alternatives such as the utilization of the Fasting Hyperglycaemia Study[22]. The role of pharmacological intervention in the prevention of type 2 diabetes remains the subject of investigation[23].

The prevention of type 2 diabetes still has numerous ambiguities, but prudent optimism must guide all our actions[1,21,24].

7.6 DIFFICULTIES AND WEAKNESSES IN THE PREVENTION OF DIABETES

A summary of the principal obstacles in the way of the prophylaxis of diabetes mellitus, as they stand at the end of the twentieth century, is given in Table 7.1.

I believe that this list must begin with the difficulties in the scientific field. Thus, with all the progress made in the last years, the genetic basis of diabetes is not yet perfectly clarified even for type 1 diabetes. The literature referring to environmental factors has grown a great deal; even so, we do not know completely what these factors are—and, especially, we lack important data on the real contributions of each of them. The pathogenetic mechanisms of diabetes are only partially clarified particularly those of type 2 diabetes. In consequence of all these weaknesses, the possibility of preventing human diabetes is still limited and insufficiently characterized from the scientific point of view.

The list continues with the lack of success on the field of practical prevention of diabetes. The international organizations (such as the WHO and the International Diabetes Federation) are preoccupied

Table 7.1. The principal obstacles in the prevention of diabetes mellitus

---

On the scientific plane:
  The genetic basis is still unclear
  There is as yet insufficient data about most of the risk factors
  The pathogenetic mechanisms are still only partially elucidated
  The possibilities of prevention are limited and insufficiently quantified
On the plane of practical action:
  The non-existence of a coherent international system for the prevention of
  diabetes (coordinated by the WHO and IDF)
  The lack of national programs for the prophylaxis of diabetes (with few
  exceptions)
  The lack or precariousness of local preventive programs (with some
  exceptions)
  Insufficient data regarding cost-effectiveness in diabetes prevention
On the social plane:
  Minimization of the problem by governments and other official
  decision-making organizations
  Ignorance of the problem by lay people
  Insufficient material resources (especially in developing countries)
  Cultural and educational deficiencies (general and specific)

---

with the prophylaxis of diabetes mellitus and have opened many horizons but they have not yet perfected an efficient international system for the resolution of this problem. Not even at the national level (with rare exceptions) are there real prevention projects, in spite of the fact that national programs for diabetes have been elaborated which tackle this disease in ensemble[25]. At the local level, preventive programs are lacking or insufficient. The lack of data at our disposal related to the cost:efficiency ratio in the prevention of diabetes has been underlined.

Another important category of difficulty is the social plane. There appears to be a tendency to minimize the problem of diabetes mellitus, especially with regard to its prevention, by governments and official institutions in various countries. Also, many other representatives of contemporary human society have ignored this problem. The lack of financial resources of the health systems of (but not exclusively) developing countries has been clearly felt in the domain of prophylaxis of diabetes. Similarly, the effects of cultural and educational deficiencies, which are greater in developing countries and in disadvantaged population groups, are notable.

Bearing in mind all these difficulties, it is clear that the prevention of diabetes will not make spectacular progress in the immediate future. It is also clear that our efforts must be magnified in such a way to give us reasonable hope for the next century.

REFERENCES

1. Clark Jr CM. How should we respond to the worldwide diabetes epidemic? *Diabetes Care* 1998; **21**: 475.
2. Efrat S. Prospects for gene therapy of insulin-dependent diabetes mellitus. *Diabetologia* 1998; **41**: 1401–1409.
3. Åkerblom HK, Knip M. Prevention of IDDM: strategies based on new observations of molecular pathogenesis. *Diabetologia* 1997; **40**: 743–748.
4. Friedman JE, Dohm GL, Leggett-Frazier N *et al*. Restoration of insulin responsiveness in skeletal muscle of morbidly obese patients after weight loss. *J Clin Invest* 1992; **89**: 701–705.
5. Cheţa D. Animal models of Type I (insulin-dependent) diabetes mellitus. *J Pediatr Endocrinol Metab* 1998; **11**: 11–19.
6. Mandrup-Poulsen T, Reiners JI, Andersen HU *et al*. Nicotinamide treatment in the prevention of insulin-dependent diabetes mellitus. *Diabetes Metab Rev* 1993; **9**: 295–309.
7. Heller B, Wang Z-Q, Wagner EF *et al*. Inactivation of the poly (ADP-ribose) polymerase gene affects oxygen radical and nitric oxide toxicity in islet cells. *J Biol Chem* 1997; **270**: 11176–11180.
8. Pozzilli P, Browne PD, Kolb H, The Nicotinamide Trialists. Meta-analysis of nicotinamide treatment in patients with recent-onset IDDM. *Diabetes Care* 1996; **19**: 1357–1363.
9. Herskowtz RD, Jackson RA, Soeldner JS, Eisenbarth GS. Pilot trial to prevent type 1 diabetes progression to overt IDDM despite oral nicotinamide. *J Autoimmun* 1989; **2**: 733–737.
10. Elliot RB, Chase HP. Prevention or delay of type 1 (insulin-dependent) diabetes in children using nicotinamide. *Diabetologia* 1991; **34**: 362–365.
11. Manna R, Migliore A, Martini LS *et al*. Nicotinamide treatment in subjects at high risk of developing IDDM improves insulin secretion. *Br J Clin Pract* 1997; **46**: 177–179.
12. Elliot RB, Pilcher CC, Fergusson DM, Stewart AW. A population based strategy to prevent insulin-dependent diabetes using nicotinamide. *J Pediatr Endocrinol Metab* 1996; **9**: 501–509.

13. Gale EAM, Bingley PJ. Can we prevent IDDM? *Diabetes Care* 1994; **17**: 339–344.
14. Lampeter EF. Intervention with nicotinamide in pre-type 1 diabetes: the Deutsche Nicotinamid Intervetionsstudie (DENIS). *Diabete Metab* 1993; **19**: 105–109.
15. Lampeter EF, Klinghammer A, Scherbaum WA *et al.* and the DENIS Group. The Deutsche Nicotinamide Intervention Study. An attempt to prevent type 1 diabetes. *Diabetes* 1998; **47**: 980–984.
16. Füchtenbusch M, Ziegler AG. Prophylactic Insulin Treatment in Pre-Type-1-Diabetes. In Marshall SM, Home PD, Rizza RA (eds). *The Diabetes Annual/10*. Amsterdam: Elsevier, 1996; 135–147.
17. Orban T, Jackson R. Insulin Treatment in Pre-diabetes. In Palmer JP (ed.). *Prediction, Prevention and Genetic Counseling in IDDM*. Chichester: Wiley, 1996; 273–282.
18. DPT-1 Study Group. The Diabetes Prevention Trial—Type 1 Diabetes (DPT-1): Progress Report. *Diabetologia* 1997; **40** (Suppl 1): A66.
19. Zivny JH, Kantele A, Lue C, Moldoveanu Z, Mestecky J, Elson CO. The modulation of cellular and humoral immune responses of orally given antigen by cholera toxin-B subunit in humans. *Immunol Cell Biol* 1997; **75** (Suppl 1).
20. Stern MP. Kelly West Lecture. Primary prevention of type II diabetes mellitus. *Diabetes Care* 1991; **14**: 399–410.
21. Manson JE, Spelsberg A. Primary prevention of non-insulin-dependent diabetes mellitus. *Am J Prev Med* 1994; **10**: 172–184.
22. Hammersley MS, Meyer LC, Morris RJ, Nanley SE, Turner RC, Holman RR. The Fasting Hyperglycemia Study: I. Subject identification and recruitment for a non-insulin-dependent diabetes prevention trial. *Metabolism* 1997; **46** (Suppl 1): 44–49.
23. Eriksson K-F. Future strategies for the prevention of type II diabetes. *Reducing the Burden of Diabetes J* 1998; **12**: 9–12.
24. Knowler WC, Narayan KM. Prevention of non-insulin-dependent diabetes mellitus. *Prev Med* 1994; **23**: 701–703.
25. King H, Gruber W, Lander T (eds). *Implementing National Diabetes Programmes. Report of a WHO Meeting*. Geneva: World Health Organization, 1995.

8

Insufficiently Utilized Opportunities

Brutus, thou sleep'st: awake, and see thyself

William Shakespeare

If we attempt to analyze the relationship between diabetes and the contemporary world, we shall observe that it is almost impossible to comprehend it all. The diagnosis of the disorder, its treatment and the treatment of its complications, the evaluation of epidemiologic parameters, the provision of financial resources, the industrial production of means of treatment and follow-up care, the establishment and functioning of associations between patients, physicians and nurses, related scientific research and the development of specialized literature and other sources of information are just some examples of fields which we should explore in order to uncover the numerous threads connecting diabetes with human society. Metaphorically speaking, the magnitude of the forces used by humankind to fight diabetes is truly impressive. The problems at the moment are, in my opinion, those of making diabetes prevention a priority of this battle and more efficient utilization of the resources at our disposal.

8.1   THE SCIENTIFIC SECTOR

Research on diabetes is being carried out in many countries. There are research units of variable size (institutes, centers, teams) as well as a wide range of interests (fundamental or applied; clinical, populational or experimental, etc.). Among these are some very prestigious scientific institutes in which renowned personalities work. They are well equipped and supplied with significant funds. Most of these elite institutions can be found in the USA, Western Europe, Japan, Canada and Australia. Some countries, such as Finland, have been obliged to accord great attention to diabetologic research as a result of the increased frequency of diabetes mellitus.

Diabetologic societies and scientific associations from different countries organize congresses, symposia and workshops, initiate research projects, offer grants and so on. The Annual Meeting of the American Diabetes Association, in its 58th year (last meeting Chicago, Illinois, 13–16 June 1998), represents one of the largest and most valuable scientific manifestations of contemporary diabetology (Table 8.1). Other important reunions are organized by the national associations of the United Kingdom, Germany or other countries with a tradition in diabetes research. Organizations from Eastern Europe, Latin America, Asia or other regions are also making laudable efforts. Romania is one such example. It has a functioning Society of Diabetes, Nutrition and Metabolic Diseases. It began to organize, from 1975, annual meetings initially designated Romanian Diabetology Days. Gradually, these events grew in magnitude to become a National Congress with international participation.

Scientific research related to certain aspects of diabetes mellitus, and scientific events dedicated to these aspects, are initiated not only by associations in the field of diabetology but also by those in numerous associated fields such as endocrinology, internal medicine, cardiology, ophthalmology, immunology, genetics and biochemistry. The practical connections of diabetology with most of the other medical specialties are reflected in the scientific field.

Research efforts in diabetes mellitus and related fields are strongly stimulated by prestigious international fora. For example, the European Association for the Study of Diabetes (EASD) held its 34th Annual Meeting in Barcelona, Spain, in September 1998 with approximately 10 000 participants (Table 8.1).

Table 8.1. Important scientific and professional organizations of contemporary diabetology

Name	Address	Last major scientific event*
International Diabetes Federation	1 rue Defacqz, B 1000 Brussels, Belgium	16th International Diabetes Federation Congress, Helsinki, 20–25 July 1997
European Association for the Study of Diabetes	Merovingerstrasse 29, D-40223 Düsseldorf, Germany	34th Annual Meeting of the EASD, Barcelona, Spain, 8–12 September 1998
American Diabetes Association	1660 Duke Street, Alexandria VA 22314, USA	58th Annual Meeting and Scientific Sessions, June 13–16, 1998, Chicago, Illinois

*By April 1999

The International Diabetes Federation (IDF) is the most representative scientific and professional diabetologic organization in the world, with 124 countries included in its membership[1]. Its mandate is: "to enhance the lives of people with diabetes". The central headquarters of the organization is in Brussels, Belgium (Table 8.1). IDF branches coordinate the activities in large geographic areas such as Africa, East Mediterranean and Middle East, North America, South and Central America, South East Asia and the Western Pacific. The 16th International Diabetes Federation Congress was held in Helsinki, Finland, in July 1997 and the next one will take place in 2000 in Mexico City. It is worthy of note that some associations for medium-level personnel as well as patients' organizations are included in, or affiliated to, the IDF and their activities are encouraged by its leadership (Table 8.2).

The volume of available scientific data has grown tremendously. Some of it is publicized during the scientific events also mentioned in related journals. In addition, a significant number of international and national periodicals, some of which have a wide readership as a result of their high scientific standard are in circulation (Table 8.3).

Table 8.2. The IDF leadership (after the Helsinki Congress in Finland, July 1997)

President:	Professor C Cockram, Hong Kong
Ms María L de Alva, Mexico	Ms L Etu-Seppälä, Finland
President elect:	Professor R Madan, India
Professor KGMM Alberti, UK	Professor M Massi-Benedetti, Italy
Vice-presidents:	Dr JC Mbanya, Cameroon
Mr B Allgot, Norway	Dr E Morrison, Jamaica
Professor M Arab, Egypt	Professor K Nagati, Tunisia
Professor M Berger, Germany	Dr A Perez-Comas, Puerto Rico
Professor F Bonnici, South Africa	Mr H Rivera, USA
Professor A Charca, Brazil	Professor M Silink, Australia
Professor D Chisholm, Australia	Ms L Siminerio, USA
Ms L Etu-Seppälä, Finland	Ms S Tucker, USA
Professor P Home, UK	Honorary presidents:
Professor T Johnson, Nigeria	Professor S Baba, Japan
Professor H Rivera, USA	Professor S Bajaj, India
Professor M Ruiz, Argentina	Professor J Hoet, Belgium
Dr J Skyler, USA	Professor H Keen, UK
Board of management:	Dr L Krall, USA
Ms María L de Alva, Mexico	Professor R Luft, Sweden
Professor KGMM Alberti, UK	Mr W Mayes Jr, USA
Mr B Allgot, Norway	Ms L Mellor, Australia
Mr E Bell, South Africa	Professor M Serrano-Rios, Spain
Professor A Chacra, Brazil	Professor A Samad Shera, Pakistan

Adapted from *IDF Bulletin* 1998, **43**(3)

Table 8.3. Some of the widely read journals in the field of diabetology

Journal title	Country or region of origin
Diabetes	USA
Diabetes Care	USA
Diabetologia	Europe
Diabetes Research and Clinical Practice	Japan
Diabetic Medicine	UK
Diabete et Metabolisme	France
Diabetes, Nutrition and Metabolism	Italy
Metabolism	USA

An increasing number of books dedicated to diabetes (monographs, textbooks, manuals, etc.) are issued by publishing houses of varying size in most countries of the world. Amongst the most famous texts are: *Joslin's Diabetes Mellitus* (in its 13th edition in 1994); *International Textbook of Diabetes Mellitus* (two volumes), in its 2nd edition in 1997; the textbooks edited by Pickup and Williams, Ellenberg and Rifkin, Davidson amongst others. Monographs dedicated to the prevention of diabetes have begun to increase in number. Two fundamental works in this field are worthy of mention: the WHO report of 1994 and the monograph edited by Palmer in 1996. Both were frequently cited in previous chapters.

The inclusion and spread of scientific data in the field of diabetology and other fields of medicine on the Internet and *Medline* (amongst others) has been of great value.

I cannot conclude this succinct synthesis of the scientific forces of diabetes without recalling to mind that, through the years, this sector of research has benefited from the contributions of some exceptional

Table 8.4. List of Claude Bernard Lecturers at annual EASD meetings

1969—Montpellier, De Duve C (B)	1984—London, Lefèbvre PJ (B)
1970—Warsaw, Sutherland EW (USA)	1985—Madrid, Pfeiffer EF (D)
	1986—Rome, Waldhäusl WF (A)
1971—Southampton, Derot M (F)	1987—Leipzig, Keen H (UK)
1972—Madrid, Lundbaek K (DK)	1988—Paris, Deckert T (DK)
1973—Brussels, Renold AE (CH)	1989—Lisbon, Tchobroutsky G (F)
1974—Jerusalem, Fraser TR (UK)	1990—Copenhagen, Alberti KGMM (UK)
1975—Munich, Spiro RG (USA)	
1976—Helsinki, Hers HG (B)	1991—Dublin, Shafrir E (IL)
1977—Geneva, Coleman DL (USA)	1992—Prague, Bennett PH (USA)
1978—Zagreb, Cruetzfeld W (D)	1993—Istanbul, Andreani D (I)
1979—Vienna, Pyke DA (UK)	1994—Düsseldorf, Reaven G (USA)
1980—Athens, Unger RH (USA)	1995—Stockholm, Berger M (D)
1981—Amsterdam, Meyer-Schwickerath GRE (D)	1996—Vienna, Ward J (UK)
	1997—Helsinki, Mogensen CE (DK)
1982—Budapest, Mirouze J (F)	
1983—Oslo, Hellerström C (S)	1998—Barcelona, Wollheim C (CH)

Adapted from the Final Programme, EASD 1998, Barcelona

personalities. Some of these have been honored by the EASD, ADA and the IDF. Table 8.4 lists the winners the Claude Bernard Medal (offered by the EASD) and Table 8.5 gives the Banting Medal Recipients (in the ADA). Some of these names later became part of the list of Nobel laureates in medicine.

Table 8.5. List of Banting Medal recipients during annual ADA meetings

1941—Joslin EP	1968—Colwell AR
1942—Muhlberg W	1969—Sutherland EW
1943—Hipwell F	1970—Lacy PE
1944—Rowtree LG	1971—Cahill GF
1946—25th Anniversary of Insulin Program:	1972—Hodgkin DC
Barach JH	1973—Lazarow A
Houssay BA	1974—Renold AE
Hagedorn HC	1975—Unger RH
Lawrence RD	1976—Steiner DF
Opie E	1977—Kipnis DM
University of Toronto	1978—Fajans SS
1947—Clowes GHA	1979—Park CR
1948—Woodyatt RT	1980—Freinkel N
1949—Evans HM	1981—Orci L
1950—Young FG	1982—Roth J
1951—Long CNH	1983—Rubenstein AH
1952—Bensley RR	1984—Foster DW
1953—Warren S	1985—Nerup B
1954—Dale HH	1986—Winegrad AI
1955—Cori CF	1987—Larner J
1956—Stadie WC	1988—Reaven GM
1957—Sterren D Jr	1989—Rosen O
1958—Conn JW	1990—Porte D
1959—Thorn GW	1992—Vranic M
1961—Levine R	1993—Kahn CR
1962—Hastings AB	1994—Cryer PE
1963—Houssay BA	1995—Matschinsky FM
1964—Annual Meeting canceled, IDF/Toronto	1996—Bennet PH
1965—Berson SA	1997—Cherrington AD
1966—Williams RH	1998—Olefsky JM
1967—Marble A	

Adapted from *Diabetes* 1998; **47** (Suppl 1): 8

8.2 THE PROFESSIONAL MEDICAL SECTOR

The army of people involved in the diagnosis, treatment and follow-up care of individuals affected with diabetes is difficult to estimate at a planetary level.

The personnel involved in primary healthcare play a major role. The diagnosis of new cases of diabetes occurs frequently at this level. This part of the medical world is also responsible for a considerable proportion of the present care of diabetic patients. It is natural that it should be so, bearing in mind the fact that it is the largest medical compartment and closest to the people; it may be considered the base of the medical pyramid. The WHO insists on an increasing involvement of primary healthcare providers in the care of type 2 diabetes mellitus, the explosive increase in which has been underlined from the beginning of this book. The putting into practice of the WHO recommendation requires—differing from country to country and from region to region—certain organizational and educational measures. It would be very useful for the stimulation, in parallel, of some preventive activity.

The specialized network that caters for the difficult problems of diabetology comprises consulting rooms, centers, departments, hospitals, university clinics, and institutes or other larger or smaller units. As well as doctors and middle level personnel, laboratory staff and people involved in ophthalmology, cardiology, surgery, neurology, nephrology participate in diabetes care. To these are added the efforts of pharmacists, chiropodists and psychologists.

The background of diabetologists differs. In many countries they are drawn from the fields of endocrine and metabolic diseases; in others they originate from the large field of internal medicine. Finally, there is also a tendency for the formation of specialists in diabetes, nutrition and metabolic diseases.

The presence of diabetologists is not, however, necessary—or even possible—everywhere. In smaller communities where the number of patients is relatively reduced, their care is usually in the hands of internists or pediatricians.

At the recommendation of the WHO, this army is restructuring its activity to conform with the provisions of national diabetes programs[2]. In Europe, the St Vincent Declaration, enunciated in 1989, is of exceptional importance (Table 8.6). It contains a number

Table 8.6. Diabetes Care and Research in Europe: The Saint Vincent Declaration (1989)

Selected five-year outcome targets
- To ensure that *care for children* with diabetes is provided by individuals and teams specialized in the management both of diabetes and of children, and that families with a diabetic child get the necessary social, economic and emotional support.
- To implement effective measures for the prevention of costly *complications*:
    Reduce new *blindness* due to diabetes by one-third or more
    Reduce the numbers of people entering end-stage diabetic *renal failure* by at least one-third
    Reduce by one-half the rate of limb amputations or diabetic *gangrene*
    Cut morbidity and mortality from *coronary heart disease* in the diabetic by vigorous programmes of risk factor reduction
    Achieve *pregnancy outcome* in the diabetic woman that approximates that of the nondiabetic women.
- Establish *monitoring and control systems* using state-of-the-art information technology for quality assurance of diabetes healthcare provision and for laboratory and technical procedures in diabetes diagnosis, treatment and self-management.

Adapted from reference 3

Table 8.7. International meeting in Lisbon (1997) to review the progress of the St Vincent Declaration

---

DIABETES CARE AND RESEARCH IN EUROPE
Fourth Meeting for the Implementation of the St Vincent Declaration
IMPROVEMENT OF DIABETES CARE
Lisbon, 26 February–1 March 1997
- Total number of countries: 56 (Seven from outside the European Region)
- Total participants: 768
- At the end of the reunion, the adoption was approved of:
    The Lisbon Statement

Adapted from the *St Vincent Declaration Newsletter* 1997, issue 11 of general objectives such as medical, social and organizational, research and diabetes care goals. To these are added precise, evidence-based achievable targets for health improvement, including the reduction by at least one-third of new cases of blindness and of development of renal failure due to diabetes, the halving of diabetes-related amputation rates, the reduction of ischemic heart disease and stroke and the normalization of pregnancy outcome[3,4]. The Declaration was endorsed by national governments in Europe at a regional World Health Assembly in 1990. The St Vincent initiative has been re-evaluated on a periodic basis. Contributions of indubitable value were made on the occasion of the last two reunions (Athens 1995, Lisbon 1997) (Table 8.7). A comprehensive assessment is expected in 1999 in Istanbul on the occasion of the tenth anniversary of the Declaration. The theme of this meeting will be "Health for all in Diabetes". In Table 8.8 there is a list of the St Vincent Working Groups, subdivided by area of interest.

Other international documents somewhat similar to the St Vincent Declaration involve other areas of the world or childhood diabetes. One example is the Declaration of the Americas on Diabetes, adopted in 1996 in San Juan, Puerto Rico[5]. All of these together have the remarkable effect of mobilization of forces and resources for the fight against diabetes mellitus.

8.3 THE SOCIAL SECTOR

Patients' organizations are more numerous and stronger than before. Some have a long tradition of producing educational brochures and journals and provide their members with moral and material support. Some bodies have been accepted in the IDF, which is a recognition and a stimulus. Unfortunately, their activities are occasionally over-shadowed by quarrels, misunderstandings and unjustifiable rivalry.

There are also charitable societies and groups whose interest in the problems of diabetics is continuously increasing. Some foundations have considerable financial resources and contribute generously in many directions to supporting diabetic research in the field of diabetes.

The media is giving increasing attention to diabetes and its social and economic consequences. Their contribution to education and

Table 8.8. List of St Vincent working groups subdivided by area of interest

Education and empowerment:
  Improving education for persons with diabetes
  Empowerment: Changing the "patient" into a "person who has diabetes"
  Improving the quality of associations for people with diabetes
Quality development:
  Improving diabetes outcomes through quality management
  Improving diabetes outcomes: The role of information technology
  Confidentiality and ethics in data collection in diabetes
  Epidemiology made practical: What are the main issues?
  The role of evidence-based medicine in diabetes care
Children and adolescents:
  Improving quality of care for children and adolescents with diabetes
  Children's camps: What should they be like to maximize the benefit to participants?
Outcomes:
  Reducing blindness and eye disease in persons with diabetes
  Reducing amputations in persons with diabetes
  Improving the outcomes for persons with diabetes nephropathy
  The common enemy: Stroke and heart disease
  Optimizing outcomes of pregnancy in women with diabetes
  Well-being and quality of life for persons with diabetes: How should it be measured?
  Improving outcomes of people with diabetes: Smoking prevention and cessation
Expanding the diabetes team:
  Mobilizing primary healthcare for improved diabetes care
  Improving the quality of diabetes care: The role of the nurse in the diabetes team
  The role of nutrition in improving outcomes for persons with diabetes
  Improving diabetes care: The role of the laboratories
  The role of the pharmacists in improving outcomes for persons with diabetes
Partnership:
  The role of the payers in improving outcomes in diabetes
  The role of industry care in improving the quality of diabetes care
  The role of the media in improving outcomes of diabetes care
  The role of service organizations in improving diabetes
Implementation and future developments:
  Implementing national diabetes programmes
  The St Vincent Declaration in an international perspective
  The St Vincent Declaration action programme into the next millenium

Adapted from *The St Vincent Declaration Newsletter* 1997, issue 13 prevention is worthy of being underlined, although more could be done. It is also a fact that the articles and the interventions on radio and television made by physicians are sometimes arid and difficult to understand for the general public and this is the reason for their diminished efficiency. The successful transmission of information (by talking or writing for the layman) is a hard task for the physician. There is need for practice and talent.

In a number of countries, the church has begun to involve itself in the promotion of a healthy lifestyle and in the prevention of chronic diseases, including diabetes mellitus. This is a natural tendency if one bears in mind the fact that in the fundamental books of the great religions there are many precepts and exhortations to living a balanced and nutritionally healthy life.

Schools and the army are other social institutions whose role in the promotion of health is of great importance (Table 8.9).

"World Diabetes Day" is observed on 14 November each year (the birthday of Frederick Banting). The observance of this day is a public awareness campaign, initiated by the IDF in 1991 and co-sponsored by the WHO from the onset. The theme selected for 1998 was "Diabetes and Human Rights"[6].

These have been just a few examples. The idea that I am trying to impress is that a problem as difficult as diabetes cannot be solved without concerted efforts of the whole of humanity. The personal efforts of the physician are insufficient if not accompanied by broad social support.

Table 8.9. Components of contemporary human society involved in the battle against diabetes mellitus

Patients' associations
Charitable societies and foundations
Mass media
Schools (at all levels)
The church
The army
Cultural institutions
Sport and fitness organizations

8.4 THE POLITICAL AND ADMINISTRATIVE SECTOR

The local and regional authorities, amongst whom can be found those who direct medical activities, could and should be more preoccupied by the diabetic pandemic. The allocation and utilization of resources in which these authorities are deeply involved are essential for the prevention of the chronic diseases. Just as significant is the existence of a well grounded program of action that is adapted to local and regional differences.

The national authorities, including the health ministry or its equivalent, have a decisive role. The prevention of diabetes must be coordinated and supported, in each country, by governmental and other central organizations. The ministry of health must carry out its activity according to the provisions of a well prepared prevention program based on clear and realistic objectives. It must ensure the cooperation of other ministries (finance, education, industry etc.) as well as other central institutions (universities, academies and scientific societies amongst others). It is expected that politicians and governments become increasingly conscious of the importance represented by the prevention of chronic disease for the future of their countries.

On the international scene, the indispensable contribution of the WHO to the problems of diabetes mellitus must be emphasized. The governing body consists of the ministries of health of over 190 member states and it convenes in Geneva each May at the World Health Assembly. The missions of the WHO are to provide international leadership in public health and to advise member governments on appropriate policies and strategies for health promotion and disease prevention[6]. We have discussed already the two fundamental WHO reports on diabetes mellitus (of 1980 and 1985) and the report (of 1994) dedicated to its prevention. The modernization of the criteria for diagnosis and classification of diabetes mellitus is a major preoccupation of the WHO at present[7]. To assist it in its various tasks and program activities, the WHO has developed a network of over 30 collaborating centers in the field of diabetes[7] (Table 8.10). From the information available and the accumulated experience, the WHO should play a major role in guiding and impelling programmes for the prevention of diabetes mellitus and its complications. We could ask, of course, that the WHO experts make more efforts in this direction: however, they are directed to cooperate more closely with

Table 8.10. WHO Collaborating Centers in the field of diabetes

---

Argentina:
WHO Collaborating Center for Diabetes, Research, Education and Care. CENEXA, 1900 La Plata

Australia:
WHO Collaborating Center for the Epidemiology of Diabetes Mellitus and Health Promotion for Noncommunicable Disease Control. International Diabetes Institute, Caulfield, VIC 3162

Bangladesh:
WHO Collaborating Center for Research and Training for the Prevention and Control of Diabetes Mellitus. BIRDEM, Dhaka 1000

Belgium:
WHO Collaborating Center for the Development of the Biology of the Endocrine Pancreas. Catholic University of Louvain, 1348 Louvain-la-Neuve

Canada:
WHO Collaborating Center for the Study of Atherosclerosis in Diabetes. Toronto Hospital (General Division), Toronto, Ontario M5G 2C4

Croatia:
WHO Collaborating Center for the Development of Appropriate Technology in the Control of Diabetes Mellitus. "Vuc Vrhovac" Institute, 41000 Zagreb

Cuba:
WHO Collaborating Center for Integrated Medical Care Services in Diabetes. Instituto Nacional de Endocrinologia, Havana 4

Czech Republic:
WHO Collaborating Center for the Development, Management and Evaluation of the National Diabetes Control Program. Postgraduate Medical Institute, 762 75 Zlin

Denmark:
WHO Collaborating Center for Research and Training on the Pathogenesis of Diabetes Mellitus. Steno Diabetes Center, 2820 Gentoffe

France:
WHO Collaborating Center for Coordination of and Training in Clinical Research and Epidemiology in Diabetes. INSERM-Unité 21, 94807 Villejuif and Hôtel-Dieu, 754004 Paris
WHO Collaborating Center for the Prevention and Control of Diabetes. 67000 Strasbourg

Germany:
WHO Collaborating Center for Diabetes Prevention. Heinrich Heine Univ., Medizinische Klinik, 40 001 Düsseldorf

(*continued*)

Table 8.10. (*continued*)

Israel:
   WHO Collaborating Center for the Study of Diabetes in Youth. CMCI, 49202 Petach-Tiqva
Italy:
   WHO Collaborating Center for the Improvement of Quality of Life in Diabetes According to the St Vincent Declaration. DIMISEM, 06126 Perugia
   WHO Collaborating Center for the Prevention of Diabetes-Related Blindness. Universita degli Studi di Torino, 10126 Torino
Japan:
   WHO Collaborating Center for Diabetes Treatment and Education. Diabetes Center, Kyoto 612
Jordan:
   WHO Collaborating Center for Diabetes Research, Education and Primary Health Care. National Center for Diabetes, PO Box 13165
Pakistan:
   WHO Collaborating Center for Treatment, Education and Research in Diabetes and Diabetic Pregnancies. Diabetic Association of Pakistan, Karachi 74600
Russian Federation:
   WHO Collaborating Center for Epidemiology, Care and Prevention in Diabetes. National Research Center for Endocrinology, 117036 Moscow
WHO Collaborating Center for Diabetes Education and Informatics. RAAMS, 125315 Moscow
Senegal:
   WHO Collaborating Center for the Control and Prevention of Diabetes Mellitus. Hôpital Communal Abase Ndao, B.P. 6054, Dakar
Switzerland:
   WHO Collaborating Center for Reference and Research in Diabetes Education. Hôpital Cantonal Universitaire, 1211 Geneva 14
United Kingdom:
   WHO Collaborating Centre for the Study and Control of Long-Term Complications of Diabetes Mellitus. Guy's Hospital, London SE1 9RT
   WHO Collaborating Centre for Training, Evaluation and Research in Diabetes. Medical School, Newcastle-upon-Tyne NE2 4HH
United States of America:
   WHO Collaborating Center for the Development of Integrated Primary Care Program for Community Practice. Centers for Disease Control and Prevention (K10), Atlanta, GA 30333
   WHO Collaborating Center for Diabetes Research, Information and Education. NIDDK-NIH, Bethseda, MD 20892-6600

(*continued*)

Table 8.10. (*continued*)

WHO Collaborating Center for Diabetes Education, Translation and Computer Technology. International Diabetes Center, Minneapolis, MN 55416

WHO Collaborating Center for Biostatistics in Diabetes. Center for Epidemiologic Research, Oklahoma City OK 73190

WHO Collaborating Center for the Design, Methodology and Analysis of Epidemiological and Clinical Investigations in Diabetes. NIDDKD, Phoenix, AZ 85014

WHO Collaborating Center for Diabetes Registries and Training in the Epidemiology of Diabetes Mellitus. Diabetes Research Center, Pittsburgh, PA 15213

Adapted from *IDF Bull* 1998; **43** (3)

national and local authorities. We should not forget that, in spite of its great prestige, the WHO is an institution with limited resources. Such an international institution could make recommendations and offer technical aid but cannot take the place of local, national and regional organizations in solving the practical problems of public health[8]. In the prevention of diabetes, the principal responsibilities are those of the communities and their representatives.

8.5 THE ECONOMIC SECTOR

The care of diabetic patients would not be possible without the contribution of producers and distributors of insulin, oral antidiabetics, medication for the treatment of complications, the means for metabolic self-monitoring, reagents and laboratory equipment. A considerable number of companies with thousands of employees are involved in this activity and the figures are on the increase. Some of these institutions are amongst the most unwavering supporters of research and of scientific meetings dedicated to diabetes (Table 8.11). In recent years, there has been increasing discussion of a new kind of partnership between medical staff and the pharmaceutics industry with the objective of better antidiabetic care.

Table 8.11. Corporate Partners of the IDF

Long-term contributors:
  Boehringer Mannheim GmbH
  Eli Lilly and Company
  Servier Research Group
  Novo Nordisk A/S
Lawrence circle:
  Bayer Corporation
  Boehringer Mannheim GmbH
  Eli Lilly and Company
  Glaxo Wellcome plc
  LifeScan Inc
  Novo Nordisk A/S
Mayes circle:
  Servier Research Group
Platinum corporate partners:
  Amylin Pharmaceutical Inc
  Bayer Corporation
  Boehringer Mannheim GmbH
  Becton Dickinson and Company
  F Hoffman-La Roche AG
  Glaxo Wellcome plc
  Servier Research Group
  LifeScan Inc
  Eli Lilly and Company
  Merck & Company Inc
  Nestlé
  Novo Nordisk A/S
  Pfizer International Inc
Corporate partners:
  Abbott Diagnostics GmbH
  Clinical Diagnostics Inc
  Dermagraft Joint Ventures
  Hoechst Marion Roussel, Inc
  LIPHA
  MiniMed
  Mycomed Pharma AS

Adapted from *IDF Bull* 1998; **43** (3)

8.6 TOWARDS THE UNION OF FORCES

From the preceding pages, it can be deduced that in the battle that humanity is obliged to fight against diabetes mellitus there is well coordinated and united action. Unfortunately, we must also recognize that, on the international, national and community scenes, many aspects of this battle can be criticized.

With all the progress registered to date, the action taken in the primary prevention of diabetes is insufficient. Not all the sectors mentioned are fully involved in prophylaxis. I believe that we are in the phase in which interest for the prevention of diabetes mellitus must extend from the scientific sector to the practical medical sector and—especially—to the social, political, administrative and economic sectors. Without a major contribution on their part, the development of the diabetes pandemic cannot be checked (Figure 8.1).

Another weak point that needs to be addressed is the insufficient coordination of efforts. The initiatives taken in different countries or regions are usually isolated, without taking into consideration similar initiatives in other areas. Their efficiency is thus reduced. The establishment of an international forum could be considered with a view to guiding and bringing to light the principal activities related to the prevention of diabetes, especially those that are practical—there are enough precedents in other fields of contemporary medicine.

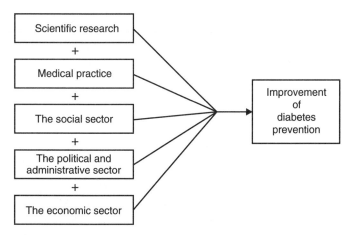

Figure 8.1. The union of the efforts aimed at better prophylaxis of diabetes mellitus

There is one more suggestion, connected with the above—the improvement of communications. The results, good or bad, of studies, as well as ideas and any other information of any sort must be circulated with more consistency all over the world. The prevention of diabetes is a major problem of the entire planet and not just of some specialized groups.

REFERENCES

1. Etu-Seppälä L. The diabetes movement: towards a better future. *IDF Bull* 1998; **43**: (3) 5–6.
2. Reiber G, King H (eds). *Guidelines for the Development of a National Programme for Diabetes Mellitus*. Geneva: World Health Organization, 1991.
3. Krans HMJ, Porta M, Keen H (eds). *Diabetes Care and Research in Europe: The St Vincent Declaration Action Programme*. Copenhagen: WHO/IDF Europe, 1997.
4. Keen H, Home PD. Organization of Care: Europe and the St Vincent Declaration Initiative. In Alberti KGMM, Zimmet P, DeFronzo RA, Keen H (eds). *International Textbook of Diabetes Mellitus*, 2nd ed. Chichester: Wiley & Sons, 1997; 1709–1717.
5. Declaration of the Americas on Diabetes. *IDF Bull* 1997; **43** (3): 12–13.
6. King H. The World Health Organization: an essential partner. *IDF Bull* 1998; **43** (3): 13–16.
7. Alberti KGMM, Zimmet PZ for the WHO Consultation. Definition, diagnosis and classification of diabetes mellitus and its complications. Part 1: diagnosis and classification of diabetes mellitus. Provisional report of a WHO consultation. *Diabetic Med* 1998; **15**: 539–553.
8. Editorial. WHO: where there is no vision, the people perish. *Lancet* 1997; **350**: 749.

Final Remarks
and Conclusions

Diabetes mellitus has become a real burden on human society at the end of the second millennium[1,2]. Population-based studies drawn from fairly complete registers of people with diabetes have shown that the costs of treatment are usually double the originally quoted figure and are almost 10% of healthcare expenditure[3,4]. How this financial burden can be reduced is becoming an increasing preoccupation of the international medical community and of the general public. Many proposals have been put forward to achieve this but they have been mostly targeted at overt diabetes and its complications. Home and Keen have emphasized the fact that resources for health are finite. How they are distributed is a global problem but preventive diabetes care is, curiously, underfunded nearly everywhere. Paradoxically, funds for "salvage therapy" of diabetes complications are often much more available[4].

The main purpose of this book has been to demonstrate that reconsideration, extension and reinforcement of primary prevention are essential to the reduction of the burden of diabetes.

Of the recent new theoretical and practical contributions which could ensure the prophylaxis of diabetes, one must mention improved diagnostic criteria and, especially, proposals for a modern etiological classification[5,6].

On the whole, new insights in the field of etiopathogenesis as well as the concepts which they have generated, have moved diabetes prevention from the field of speculation to that of projects and programs. This is already a major step forward.

The greatest problems are in prevention of type 2 diabetes mellitus. In 1996, it was estimated that type 2 diabetes affected 110 million people worldwide and more than 215 million are expected to be afflicted with this disorder by the 2010. Furthermore, half of these cases will remain undiagnosed[2]. However, there is increasing evidence that type 2 diabetes is a preventable disease. Intensive dietary regulation and increased physical activity are now established as the basic intervention approaches in IGT as well as in early type 2 diabetes. These approaches should also be recommended in populations with a high incidence of type 2 diabetes and in individuals with a family history of diabetes. Unfortunately, compliance with a long-term diet and exercise program may be difficult to achieve in many settings. The role of pharmacological intervention in the prevention of type 2 diabetes remains to be investigated[7].

Type 1 diabetes mellitus is considered a chronic disorder that results from autoimmune destruction of the insulin-producing pancreatic beta cells. Studies using animal models (NOD mice and BB rats) have suggested many interesting possibilities for preventive action. Some of these (such as nicotinamide and insulin) are already in use, with varying degrees of efficiency, in trials on human subjects.

A better correlation of all social forces involved in combating diabetes is a *sine qua non* for its prevention.

REFERENCES

1. Roman SH, Harris MI. Management of diabetes mellitus from a public health perspective. *Curr Ther Diabetes* 1997; **26**: 443–474.
2. Rabasa-Lhoret R, Chiasson J-L. Failure to treat Type II diabetes and its consequences. *Reducing the Burden of Diabetes J* 1998; **12**: 5–8.
3. Currie CJ, Kraus D, Morgan CL, Gill L, Stott NC, Peters JR. NHS acute sector expenditure for diabetes: The present, future and excess in-patient cost of care. *Diabetic Med* 1997; **14**: 686–692.
4. Home P, Keen H. Making progress with diabetes care: A story from the United Kingdom. *IDF Bull* 1998; **43** (3): 8–12.

5. The Expert Committee on the Diagnosis and Classification of Diabetes Mellitus. Report of the Expert Committee on the Diagnosis and Classification of Diabetes Mellitus. *Diabetes Care* 1997; **20**: 1183–1197.
6. Alberti KGMM, Zimmet PZ for the WHO Consultation. Definition, diagnosis and classification of diabetes mellitus and its complications. Part 1: Diagnosis and classification of diabetes mellitus. Provisional report of a WHO consultation. *Diabetic Med* 1998; **15**: 539–553.
7. Eriksson K-F. Future strategies for the prevention of type II diabetes. *Reducing the Burden of Diabetes J* 1998; **12**: 9–12.

Index

Note: numbers indexed in **bold** refer to figures or tables

mucosal surfaces, NOD mice, 91
multiple sclerosis, oral antigen
tolerization, 82
mumps
environmental factors, 146
type 1 diabetes, 26
Mycobacterium tuberculosis, type 1
diabetes in animal models, 49
myocardial ischemia, diabetes and,
3

National Institutes of Health,
impaired glucose tolerance (IGT),
119–20
neuropathy, diabetic, 3
New Zealand white rabbit, type 1
diabetes, 45
nicotinamide, type 1 diabetes
prevention, 67–71
in animals, 53
in humans, 147–8
nicotinamide adenine dinucleotide
(NAD), type 1 diabetes, 68
NIDDM, *see* type 2 diabetes
nitric oxide, beta cells and autoimmune attack, 57
nitrosamines, type 1 diabetes, 28, 66
NOD (non-obese diabetic) mouse
CTB-insulin, 86, 90
oral antigen tolerization, 84–6
oral insulin tolerization, **91**
protamine zinc insulin, 75
type 1 diabetes, 45, 46–57
Nurses' Health Study, USA
nutrition and, 122
physical activity and, 127
nutrition, 49
type 1 diabetes, 28–9, 49
type 2 diabetes, 102, 103, 121–4

obesity
in type 2 diabetes, 103, 121–4

see also body mass index (BMI);
physical activity
OGTT, impaired glucose tolerance
(IGT), 120
OM-89, 87
animal models, 85, 86
oral antigen tolerization, type 1
diabetes, 80–91, 147
oral drug failure, 14
oral insulin tolerization, NOD mice,
91
oral tolerance study, European,
88–91
orlistat, type 2 diabetes, 123
osteoporosis, physical activity and,
125
Otsuka Long Evans Tokushima Fatty
(OLETF) rat
physical activity and, 126
type 2 diabetes, 122

pancreas, in type 2 diabetes, 108,
108
pancreatectomy, 44
pathogenesis, type 2 diabetes, 105–7
pathogenic mechanisms, type 1
diabetes, 23–34
PATHWAYS weight loss program,
type 2 diabetes, 123
patients (Bucharest, 1984)
general features of, **12**
questionable insulin dependency,
15
type 1 diabetes, **14**
without insulin therapy, **13**
pellagra, type 1 diabetes prevention,
67
pentamidine, type 1 diabetes, 28
pentoxifylline, type 1 diabetes
prevention in animals, 54
peripheral vascular disease, diabetes
and, 3

Index compiled by A.C. Purton